THE BOOK
OF
Sleep

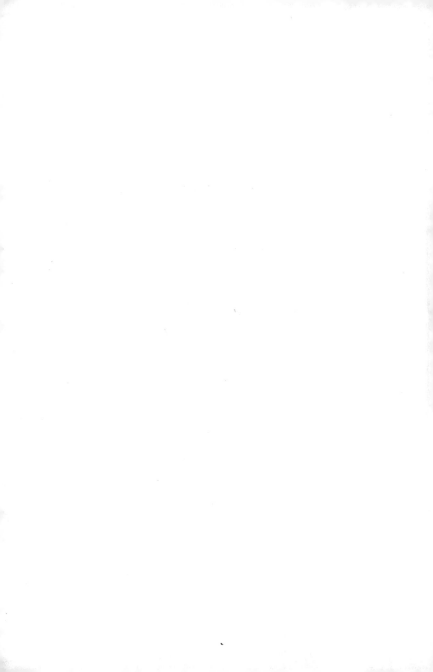

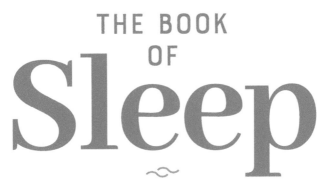

THE BOOK OF Sleep

75 STRATEGIES TO RELIEVE INSOMNIA

Dr. Nicole Moshfegh, PsyD

ROCKRIDGE
PRESS

Interior and Cover Designer: Amanda Kirk
Photo Art Director/Art: Janice Ackerman
Editor: Lia Ottaviano
Production Editor: Edgar Doolan
Cover Photo: © 2019 iPhotoDesign/Shutterstock
Author Photo: Courtesy of © 2019 Jason Miyashiro

ISBN: Print 978-1-64152-791-0 | eBook 978-1-64152-792-7

To Salar,

my best friend, partner,
and endless supporter.

Contents

Introduction:
Tired but Wired!

N ot getting the sleep you need is a univer-
sally frustrating experience. Perhaps
you're here because you can relate,
and you're desperately searching for ways to get
better sleep.

You are not alone.

Millions of individuals experience insomnia and
other sleep difficulties. But the good news is we now
have decades of research on natural, drug-free techniques scientifically proven to help you sleep better
with practice, patience, and time.

As a clinical health psychologist and insomnia
specialist, I have over a decade of training and
experience helping hundreds of individuals overcome sleep difficulties and boost their overall
well-being. Although insomnia has been on the rise,
there's a shortage of healthcare professionals with
sufficient training and expertise in sleep disorders.
For physicians, this is usually because they have
so much they're already learning about the human

body in medical school, and they only receive a few cursory lectures on sleep. In conjunction with the unique stressors of our modern society, this lack of expertise has contributed to a growing epidemic of sleepless people in search of the right help, but unable to find it. Many have come to see me after experiencing insomnia for years on end, often trying every pill imaginable and at their wits' end. I have also seen all these individuals improve their sleep once offered the correct tools and understanding.

My goal in writing this book is to also provide *you* with the education and skills necessary to work through your insomnia and finally get the sleep you've been longing for. With simple strategies based on thousands of research studies, clinical trials, and my own experience in treating individuals with insomnia, you, too, can tackle your sleep difficulties in a matter of a few weeks to months. A well-rested you is on the horizon.

Getting Started

In this section, you'll learn more about the definition and widespread prevalence of insomnia, the long-term impacts of untreated cases, and how the strategies in this book can assist you in alleviating your symptoms. I will also cover how to best use this book in order to achieve optimal relief.

IF YOU ARE CURRENTLY EXPERIENCING INSOMNIA, it's likely that you've been struggling to find a solution for some time now. The road to recovery can sometimes be a frustrating process with many ups and downs. Any setbacks you might experience while addressing your symptoms are normal—keep that in mind so you don't get discouraged. Keep trying, be patient, and treat yourself with kindness throughout this process.

Before moving forward, I would like you to take a few seconds to acknowledge, congratulate, and thank yourself for taking this first big step toward achieving natural insomnia relief. I'm glad you're here. Now, let's dive in together and find out more about how you can take control of your sleep and establish a well-balanced life.

YOU'RE NOT ALONE

When you're suffering from symptoms of insomnia, it can indeed feel like you are alone in your pain. This can cause you to feel isolated and cut off from the joys of life, contributing to feelings of hopelessness that you will ever be able to feel "normal" again. If you can relate, it's important to know that at any given moment, there are millions of people feeling the exact way you do.

In fact, one in every three adults suffers from symptoms of insomnia—that's over eighty million people in the United States alone! It's estimated that about 6% to 10% of individuals meet criteria for an insomnia disorder and up to 20% of people report significant insomnia symptoms during primary care visits. Even among those who don't meet the diagnostic criteria for an insomnia disorder, many experience daytime impairments like distress and fatigue due to their symptoms.

To be diagnosed with an insomnia disorder, you need to be subjectively (or, in other words, in your *perception*) dissatisfied with either the quantity or quality of your sleep. This can manifest in different ways, from difficulty falling asleep (known as sleep-onset or initial insomnia), difficulty staying asleep (known as sleep maintenance or middle insomnia), waking up earlier than you intended and not being able to get back to sleep (known as late insomnia), or consistently experiencing nonrestorative or non-restful sleep, despite having an adequate opportunity to sleep.

Insomnia is classified as a sleep-*wake* disorder, meaning that experiencing dissatisfaction with sleep also causes people to experience distress or impairment while they're awake. This can take on many forms, such as constantly feeling tired or fatigued, calling in sick from school or work, or experiencing difficulty concentrating on or initiating tasks. It can also cause physical and mental health symptoms such as a low mood, irritability, anxiety, worry, lower frustration tolerance, headaches, muscle aches, stomach upsets, and so on.

In order to meet criteria for an insomnia disorder, these sleep difficulties need to occur for at least three months or longer—otherwise known as **chronic** or **persistent insomnia**.

When brief periods of insomnia lasting *less* than three months are accompanied by significant distress or are interfering with a person's social, personal, academic, or occupational functioning, it is classified as **situational** or **acute insomnia**.

Because acute insomnia usually resolves without intervention, many of the evidence-based treatments currently available were developed to treat chronic insomnia. When insomnia persists for longer than a few months, it usually takes on a life of its own—whatever it was that initially triggered the insomnia is not what causes it to persist. Instead, there are several other perpetuating factors we need to examine: your circadian clock, sleep drive, and arousal disruptors. If we can change these through behavioral and cognitive interventions, sleep will improve.

Keep in mind that certain strategies will be more relevant to your situation than others. Rest assured that whether you are experiencing acute, chronic, mild, moderate, or severe symptoms, this book will provide you with a multitude of options to address your specific sleep issues.

After witnessing the immense relief my clients experience when they better understand what triggered their insomnia and what causes it to persist, and guiding them through developing a plan to address their symptoms, I know that the strategies in this book work. I have no doubt that with time, you, too, can be one of the countless individuals who experience relief from their symptoms and get back to the joys of life.

INSOMNIA IN THE LONG TERM

I f you're reading this book, you are already on the path toward reducing your insomnia symptoms. But sometimes, your journey may not be so straightforward. Speedbumps are a normal part of any change-related process, but not addressing your insomnia symptoms (or addressing them in harmful ways like with alcohol or pills) can potentially lead to detrimental health consequences in the long run.

Before we discuss the research on the specific health consequences of untreated insomnia, please know that my goal is not to add to any feelings of anxiety you may already be experiencing surrounding the impacts of your symptoms. If you experience too much anxiety or distress while reading this section (or even after reading the previous sentence), I suggest that you skip this section for now and move on to page 12 to read about how the strategies in this book can help you.

Although it can be overwhelming to read about some of these consequences, it can also be a helpful reminder that the challenges you might experience when initially implementing some of these strategies will pay off in the long run.

There has been a great deal of emphasis placed on the impacts of sleep deprivation in media and news outlets in recent years. While much of that information has been useful in educating the general public and those who purposefully deprive themselves of sleep (or who are placed in unhealthy work environments), it has inadvertently contributed to increased anxiety for insomnia sufferers, further escalating the problem. Keep in mind that much of the research on the long-term consequences of untreated insomnia or sleep deprivation has been conducted on individuals who have experienced years and years of very severe suffering. And while you may fall into that camp, it is important to know that many of these risk factors and health consequences can be reversed once you experience relief from your symptoms. Additionally, some of the health consequences popularized by the media do not always cite studies that uphold rigorous scientific standards. I hope to dispel any myths you may have heard about insomnia consequences by providing you with the most up-to-date and well-researched facts.

If an insomnia disorder is left untreated, it can lead to the later development of additional mental health symptoms and disorders, including depressive disorders, anxiety and substance use disorders, and post-traumatic stress disorder if the individual has also experienced a trauma in the course of their illness. Insomnia has also been shown to predict suicide. Additionally, if an individual already has a preexisting depressive disorder, insomnia can make it more difficult for the individual to recover from their depression. And, if the individual does recover from their depression but their insomnia symptoms linger, it can leave them more vulnerable to experiencing depression again in the future.

Untreated insomnia disorders can also impact the way our heart, blood vessel system, metabolism, and thought processes function. In particular, those who have been experiencing insomnia for at least one year, and who frequently receive less than five hours per night of sleep on average, are at increased risk of high blood pressure and type 2 diabetes. Chronic and severe insomnia is also associated with an increased risk of experiencing a heart attack. The research indicates that these illnesses potentially develop over time due to the activation of the stress system and inflammation process that occurs when an individual is chronically sleep deprived.

In terms of thought processes, individuals with insomnia can sometimes experience increased difficulty with taking the time to think before acting on something, to tackle new or unanticipated challenges, to think about things in more than one way, or to resist temptations or ignore distractions. There is some variability and discrepancy across studies conducted on executive functioning in individuals with insomnia, with some people experiencing minimal to no impairment, so these results should be interpreted with caution. In addition, individuals with chronic insomnia (as well as other sleep problems) are at higher risk for developing Alzheimer's disease, a neurodegenerative disorder that progressively destroys memory and thinking skills.

From a functional and societal standpoint, untreated insomnia can also leave an individual at increased risk for absenteeism as well as reduced productivity at work and an overall reduced quality of life.

Although there are many potential long-term health and functional consequences for untreated insomnia and sleep deprivation in general, the good news is you're taking steps toward addressing your symptoms now, so you'll be able to help prevent many of these health issues from developing in the future.

HOW THESE STRATEGIES CAN HELP

Although there are a wide array of pharmacologic and non-pharmacologic interventions available to treat insomnia, one class of interventions has proven itself to be the most effective—Cognitive Behavioral Therapy, or CBT.

CBT, pioneered by Drs. Aaron T. Beck and Albert Ellis, adheres to the basic premise that psychological or emotional distress is maintained not just by behavioral factors, but also by the unhelpful ways we think about our problems. CBT teaches people better ways of coping with their difficulties through modifying these faulty thoughts and behaviors.

Most people think of insomnia as solely a medical or physical health problem. But the truth is our minds and bodies are strongly interconnected. Even the leading causes of death, such as heart disease, dementia, diabetes, or cancer, have all been linked to chronic stress or psychological difficulties, highlighting the importance of both medical *and* psychological intervention or prevention efforts for these illnesses. Insomnia is no exception.

While insomnia can occasionally have an insidious onset without an easily identifiable trigger, most of the time there is some stressor that precipitates it. But the factors that initially contribute to the development of insomnia are not what maintain it. Instead, there are only three factors that cause insomnia to persist—disruptions in our circadian clock, our sleep drive, and our arousal system (e.g., chronic levels of stress or anxiety around sleep). When an individual experiences insomnia symptoms for longer than several months, it often causes them to turn to behaviors that they think will help them cope, like staying in bed longer after constantly waking up in the middle of the night. But these only cause the problem to worsen and persist. Cognitive and behavioral factors such as unhealthy sleeping patterns or habits can cause disruptions in any of these three perpetuating factors. CBT strategies focus on cognitions and behaviors as targets of change.

While CBT can be used to treat a variety of disorders, a specific type of CBT, known as CBT for Insomnia (or CBT-I), was developed for the exclusive purpose of treating insomnia. Across numerous research studies, CBT-I has proven to be effective in treating adults with chronic insomnia. In fact, the American College of Physicians, the largest medical-specialty organization and second-largest physician group in the United States, has even recommended that all adults receive CBT-I as the initial treatment for chronic insomnia (before medication), stating that "CBT-I provides better overall value than pharmacologic treatment."

The main strategies used in CBT-I include education on sleep and sleep hygiene, sleep (or time in bed) restriction therapy, stimulus control therapy, cognitive therapy, and various counter-arousal methods.

Sleep hygiene provides individuals with the necessary components to achieve better sleep. Sleep hygiene can be thought of like flossing, although it is a necessary component to preventing gum disease or tooth decay, you still need to brush your teeth regularly and receive the appropriate treatment if a disease develops. Because sleep hygiene is a necessary but not sufficient part of tackling your insomnia, the other strategies are also used.

Sleep restriction works by initially reducing the amount of time you spend in bed in order to increase your sleep drive and ability to sleep soundly throughout the night, while **stimulus control** breaks a learned association between your bed and not sleeping. Depending on your unique situation, you may use just one method or both methods together.

The **counter-arousal methods** primarily used in CBT-I include cognitive therapy and various relaxation strategies. **Cognitive therapy** changes unhelpful thoughts about sleep that contribute to anxiety and continued sleeplessness, by teaching you how to challenge and restructure faulty thoughts. Relaxation strategies such as progressive muscle relaxation, diaphragmatic breathing, and imagery training, reduce physiological arousal by helping to relax our "fight-or-flight" response (otherwise known as the sympathetic nervous system). They allow our rest system (the parasympathetic nervous system) to do its job, which is necessary for sleep.

Although CBT-I has been considered the "gold standard" of insomnia treatments for several years, there is burgeoning evidence for the use of various mind-body therapies in the treatment of insomnia as well. In particular, mindfulness meditation, tai chi, qigong, and yoga have all been well researched and proven to reduce insomnia symptoms. Mind-body therapies work to alleviate insomnia symptoms by reducing physiological arousal, much like relaxation. While there is growing evidence that these forms of mind-body treatments can improve insomnia symptoms on their own, they are mostly used in conjunction with the traditional CBT-I strategies just described, especially in the case of chronic and more severe insomnia.

Thousands of clinical trials have proven their effectiveness, but I've also seen them work firsthand in my experience in treating insomnia sufferers. The strategies in this book all draw from CBT-I, relaxation, and mind-body therapies in order to provide you with a wide array of the best available strategies to achieve relief from your symptoms.

MAKING THE MOST OF THIS BOOK

Now that you know more about insomnia and the evidence-based treatments for it, it's time for you to identify and learn about the different ways you can personally achieve lasting relief. In the chapters to follow, you will find seventy five different strategies, all chosen because of their effectiveness in providing you with maximal relief from your symptoms—proven through the best available research.

While there are many books available on the treatment of insomnia, what makes this book unique is that it does not adhere to a one-size-fits-all approach. Our lived experiences, background, environment, and culture all work to shape who we are, how we view the world and relate to others, and even the manner in which different health symptoms develop and persist. It is impossible for there to be just one strategy or one "formula" that will work for every person on this planet. For this reason, I have provided you with a variety of options to choose from in order to create an optimal plan that best suits you and your unique needs.

While this book is designed so that you can easily identify which strategy or strategies work best for you simply by looking through the table of contents and flipping to the page that explains how to implement your strategy of choice and why it works, sometimes it can still be overwhelming to know where to start and how to keep going. Therefore, I am also providing you with some general guidelines that will help you make the most of this book by identifying your best plan. Keep in mind that this book is also designed to be used in conjunction with any existing therapeutic treatment you are already receiving, from medication to psychotherapy.

I recommend that you first start with identifying which perpetuating factors (sleep drive, clock, or arousal disruptors) are causing your insomnia to persist. This is best accomplished by keeping a sleep diary for at least one week before you dive into implementing the other strategies in this book. Sleep diaries can help us recognize patterns or behaviors we may not be aware of that are contributing to our symptoms. You can find out how to do this by reading "Keep a Sleep Diary" on page 21. I also recommend that you continue to keep a sleep diary while implementing the other strategies in this book to enable you to track your progress.

After you have completed a diary for at least one to two weeks to establish your baseline, it is time for you to make sense of what you recorded. This will allow you to more easily identify the strategies that best pertain to your unique situation. You can accomplish this by reading "Increase Your Insight" on page 31.

Once you have identified your perpetuating factors, you're ready to start implementing sleep hygiene rules by using the "Sleep Hygiene" sidebar on page 36. These sleep hygiene strategies will be your basics.

After you have put all of your sleep hygiene rules in place, you can focus on resolving your other perpetuating factors. Move on to implementing the strategies that address sleep drive and/or biological clock disruptors, taken from "Increase Your Insight," on pages 33–34, and put them into your action plan from the "Make an Action Plan" sidebar on page 48.

While some will experience relief just from following the above steps, most of the time you will still need to add at least one or two counter-arousal strategies into your plan. That's why, outside of what I've just outlined, counter-arousal strategies make up the rest of this book. You will receive a plethora of options (forty to be exact) to reduce your arousal, provide you with additional information, identify workarounds if something has not been feasible or successful for you, provide encouragement, and troubleshoot any difficulties you might experience throughout this process.

Insomnia is a debilitating and sometimes life-threatening illness that can impact many areas of your life. After being on the recovery journey with countless individuals suffering not only from sleep issues, but also a variety of other mental health difficulties and life stressors, I acutely feel and understand the pain and struggle. I know how easy it can be to lose hope. But I've also had the privilege of being present with people who thought there was no end in sight, but come out on the other side happier and healthier than they ever could have imagined. This is what allows me to say with confidence that you can eventually get there as well.

So, let's take it one breath at a time, and remember that with some motivation and determination, you can change your life by improving your sleep.

Keep a Sleep Diary

WHY IT WORKS

One of the main tools we use to assess insomnia and track progress is a sleep diary—a daily log of the quantity and quality of your sleep the previous night. This allows us to more accurately recall details that will be important in addressing your insomnia. You may be tempted to use a fitness tracker (e.g., Fitbit, Apple Watch); however, these devices only detect movement, not sleep. The only way to accurately and objectively measure sleep is through polysomnography, or an overnight sleep study. But insomnia isn't objective. Insomnia is about our *subjective* experience of sleep—how we think we are sleeping—which is why a sleep diary is especially useful.

HOW TO DO IT

Every morning, record your previous night's sleep using the chart on the next page:

	TODAY'S DATE *Example:* 7.8.19
What time did you get in bed yesterday?	11 p.m.
What time did you try to go to sleep?	11:30 p.m.
How long did it take you to fall asleep?	1 hour
How many times did you wake up throughout the night? How long did they last in total?	2 times, total of 1.5 hours
What time was your final awakening? Was this earlier than you intended?	6 a.m., yes
What time did you get out of bed for the day?	8 a.m.
Other Comments (naps, caffeine, exercise, illness)	Took a nap for 30 minutes at 3 p.m.

(Note: In the example above, total sleep time was 4 hours and time in bed was 8.5 hours.)

TRY IT!

Keep a diary every night for at least one to two weeks and see if you notice any patterns. The diary is meant to be an estimate—there is no need to check the clock and write notes down throughout the night, just take your best guess at answering these questions as soon as you wake up. The diary will help you determine what factors are interfering with your sleep and will help you track your progress overall.

Rhythm—You Can Feel It

WHY IT WORKS

We all have an internal body clock, otherwise known as our circadian rhythm, that helps to determine the timing of our sleep. However, our circadian rhythm is naturally longer than a twenty-four-hour day. In order for our body to manage the drift that occurs as a result of our longer rhythm, our body uses cues from our environment.

A regular rise time is one variable that helps us "set" our clock and manage this drift. If you have ever traveled from one time zone to another and experienced "jet lag," you will understand this feeling. Waking up at a different time every day can make our bodies think we are constantly traveling through time zones even though we're not. If you don't want to experience that lag, keep your rise time consistent, even on the weekends.

In order to determine a standard rise time:

1. Identify what time you would naturally get up if you didn't have a schedule.
2. Identify the earliest time you need to be up for your schedule.
3. If these times are within about an hour of each other, set your alarm somewhere between them, every day.
4. If these times are discrepant by more than one hour, then be as efficient as you can on the mornings you are required to be up earlier so that you can set your alarm at the latest time possible. Don't allow yourself to sleep in the other days; keep your rise time consistent.

Quit *Lying* to Yourself

WHY IT WORKS

Our brains are constantly working overtime. To keep our brain from getting too overloaded while remaining efficient and helping us learn, it comes up with shortcuts. One way it does this is through classical conditioning—training our brain to exhibit an *automatic* response to a stimulus. Our brain learns to pair certain objects with certain responses.

Since we all have to lie down on some sort of surface or bed to sleep, over time our brain begins to associate our bed (stimulus) with sleep (response). However, when we regularly lie awake in bed due to anxiety or trouble sleeping, our brain slowly begins to associate our bed with stress and anxiety, not sleep. The good news is you can extinguish this conditioned response, if you *quit lying* in bed when you are not sleeping.

If you have been in bed for what feels like longer than twenty minutes (just don't check that clock) and you know that sleep is nowhere on the horizon, get out of bed and go sit somewhere comfy and cozy other than your bed. Once there, do something relaxing and, ideally, slightly boring (read a non-exciting book, fold clothes, etc.) until you notice yourself feeling sleepy. Once sleepy, get back into bed and sleep. If sleep is still not coming, repeat the process. Remember, this applies to the beginning, middle, and end of your sleep time, so if you wake up earlier than you intend to, get out of bed as well.

Wind Down

WHY IT WORKS

Longer work hours and constant exposure to light and technology have made it harder for us to give ourselves a mental break and unwind from the day. This contributes to an arousal overload, which can make it impossible for us to fall asleep, stay asleep, or get restorative sleep. It can be hard to remind ourselves that getting back to finishing that work project, studying for that exam, or scrolling through our social media feed right before we get in bed for the night does not allow our body enough time to calm down. You wouldn't expect a child to go from running around and watching their favorite show to falling asleep right away. The same applies to adults. We need to give our brain a chance to unwind from the day by reducing stimulation so it knows it's time to sleep.

Get in the habit of giving yourself a cutoff time for all school/work/life-related tasks before you get into bed. Ideally, provide yourself at least one hour before your bedtime (or up to two if you are trying to get to bed earlier) of only engaging in calming, enjoyable, and relaxing activities. While it's better to avoid screens during this time, if you do use them, make sure to reduce the blue light on your devices. If you decide to watch TV or read a book, choose something that's not too stimulating or that might tempt you to "binge" watch or read.

Increase Your Insight

WHY IT WORKS

While there are many triggers for developing insomnia, there are only three that cause it to persist—a homeostatic disruption, a circadian disruption, and hyperarousal. It's important for you to understand which one(s) pertain to you to properly address your symptoms.

A homeostatic disruption occurs when there is reduced sleep drive—think of it like not having a full tank of gas to get you through the night. A circadian disruption occurs when your bedtime and rise time are too variable. Hyperarousal occurs when we have too much anxiety or stress.

HOW TO DO IT

Determine the culprit of your insomnia by asking yourself these questions:

1. Homeostatic disruption:
   a. Are you napping during the day?
   b. Are you sedentary most of the day?

     c. Are you consuming substances like caffeine, nicotine, or alcohol?

     d. Are you spending time in bed when not sleeping?

2. Biological clock:

     a. Is there an hour or more of variability in the time you wake up every day?

     b. Are you naturally a night owl trying to wake up early or vice versa?

3. Hyperarousal:

     a. Do you spend a lot of time worrying while trying to sleep?

     b. Are you worried about your sleep?

     c. Do you think it is necessary to strictly engage in particular routines/behaviors in order to fall or stay asleep?

     d. Are you anxious, frustrated, or distressed while trying to sleep?

     e. Are you chronically stressed because of work, school, or other factors?

If you answered yes to one or more questions in each section, please find the corresponding solutions for each.

Strategies Addressing Homeostatic Disruption:

PAGE #	STRATEGY NAME
40	Cannabis, Cannot Sleep?
44	Nix the Caffeine
46	You're Getting Sleepy
50	Kick That Smoking Habit
52	Reconsider That Nightcap
54	Get Your Body Moving
56	Leave Napping to Babies
69	No Pain, No Gain
87	Are You Really Sleepy?
126	Assess Your Alertness
163	Stay Awake
193	Don't Stress, Compress

Strategies Addressing Clock Disruption:

PAGE #	STRATEGY NAME
25	Rhythm—You Can Feel It
67	Birds of a Feather Sleep Together

Strategies Addressing Hyperarousal:

SLEEP HYGIENE

Sleep hygiene refers to a set of practices and habits that set the stage for receiving good sleep. Although sleep hygiene items are non-negotiables, in most cases they will rarely be sufficient in addressing your insomnia symptoms alone. They will, instead, be the foundation on which your insomnia treatment plan is built.

In the next chart, you will find a list of sleep hygiene strategies. After reviewing each strategy, return to this page and check off the strategies you are already following. Make sure to incorporate all of the strategies you did not check off into your action plan for addressing your insomnia. We will revisit how to complete your action plan later on in "Make an Action Plan" on page 48.

Schedule "Worry" Time

WHY IT WORKS

Ever noticed yourself feeling tired before you crawl in bed for the night, but as soon as your head hits the pillow, your minds starts racing? If you are prone to feeling this "switch" between feeling drowsy and feeling wide awake as soon as you get in bed, your brain is giving you signals that it's time to start planning for the next day or worrying about why in the world you are not sleeping. The problem is, not only will this build up the connection between the bed and being awake, but it also increases your level of arousal, which, in turn, overrides your brain's natural ability to produce sleep. It's better to get in the habit of planning or worrying hours before you get into bed to both give your brain time to unwind from the day as well as break that bed-worry association.

Get in the habit of scheduling regular time to plan or even worry earlier in your day. For the next two weeks, allot yourself twenty minutes to write out your to-do list or any worries that have accumulated that day. Try to do this at least two to three hours before you plan to be in bed, and ideally as soon as your required work/life-related tasks have ended for the day. If you find yourself up in bed worrying again, remind yourself that you will revisit it tomorrow during your next scheduled worry time.

Cannabis, Cannot Sleep?

WHY IT WORKS

Studies on the efficacy of cannabis in the treatment of insomnia are still in their infancy. Here's what current research has provided evidence for so far: Sleep disturbance is a known withdrawal symptom of marijuana use (even when exposed to low doses); THC is associated with daytime sleepiness, delayed sleep onset, and a decrease in slow-wave (or restorative) sleep; and any short-term benefit marijuana users may initially experience (typically decreased sleep onset) vanishes after long-term/chronic use, due to a buildup of tolerance. Moreover, there are several studies also showing a strong association between heavy marijuana use and sleep disturbances.

If you have recently cut back on cannabis use and your insomnia has grown more severe, you may be experiencing withdrawal symptoms. The good news is utilizing this book can still aid you in reducing your insomnia symptoms. However, it may take you longer to see progress, so remember to be patient.

You may be tempted to begin using again because your sleep has been so poor, but this will only make your insomnia worse in the long run. Instead, try writing down the reasons why you decided to cut back and the potential benefits of your decision. Keep these nearby as reminders. Consider speaking with a trained professional or joining a support group for additional assistance.

Savor Your Bed

WHY IT WORKS

Our brains are constantly interacting with and interpreting our environment, telling us what to do next, what to feel, what to think. Have you ever experienced eating a delicious meal and then described this meal to someone else the next day while noticing your mouth begins to water? Then you understand classical conditioning—our brain's ability to pair something (an object, thought, memory, etc.) with a certain response.

If you're eating, reading, watching TV, or on your laptop, phone, or other device all while you are in bed, over time your brain most certainly begins to automatically and unconsciously pair your bed with everything *but* sleep. In fact, research shows that those who spend time in bed doing things other than sleeping are found to be poor sleepers. So let's treat our beds like that delicious meal—savoring it for sleep alone, with sex being the only exception.

Make a habit of not engaging in activities other than sleep or sex in your bed—and ideally your entire bedroom. Consider removing all distractions such as the TV, computer, and even your phone if possible. Create another comfortable area for you to engage in these activities outside of your bed/bedroom, and try to remind yourself that although this might be challenging in the beginning, you will soon reap the rewards of better sleep.

Nix the Caffeine

WHY IT WORKS

The longer we have been awake, the more our body builds up a chemical called adenosine, which is responsible for increasing our sleep signals and decreasing our wake signals. When we consume caffeine, it blocks the ability of adenosine to communicate sleep signals to our brain. Because caffeine has a half-life of five to seven hours, if you have caffeine around 7 p.m., half of it will still be in your system at 2 a.m. As soon as your body clears the caffeine out, you will "crash." So not only will that cup of coffee you drank at 7 p.m. the night before prevent you from getting adequate sleep, but by the time you start your day around 9 a.m., your sleep signals will be even stronger due to your lack of sleep and all the adenosine that was building but couldn't be released. This leads to a never-ending cycle. If you don't want to constantly time how much caffeine will still be in your body at bedtime, it's better to cut back.

It's challenging to reduce caffeine intake for many reasons, but start by trying to avoid caffeine after lunch and limiting yourself to no more than 200 to 300 mg of caffeine per day (which is roughly equivalent to two eight-ounce cups of coffee depending on the brew). Remember that decaf coffee, dark chocolate, and some pain relievers also contain caffeine.

You're Getting Sleepy

WHY IT WORKS

Insomnia can contribute to feelings of fatigue throughout the day. Many of us think if we "rest" or go to bed earlier than usual, it will give our body more opportunity to produce sleep. While this strategy may work for someone who is sleep deprived because of a lack of *opportunity* to sleep, it will generally not work if you have chronic insomnia, since you *do* have the opportunity but *can't* sleep. As counterintuitive as it may sound, resist the siren call of your pillow until you notice yourself feeling sleepy.

A person who can't sleep is already conditioned to associate the bed with being awake, so unless they are extremely sleepy, they won't fall asleep quickly, which inevitably makes problems worse. Furthermore, the more we "rest," the less opportunity our body has to build up enough sleep drive to keep us sleeping soundly throughout the night. For more on telling the difference between when you're tired versus when you're ready to sleep, see "Are You Really Sleepy?" on page 87.

HOW TO DO IT

For the next two weeks, don't get in bed just because you feel fatigued. If you absolutely feel like you need to rest, and as long as you weren't sedentary all day long, you can do so on a piece of furniture other than your bed. As soon as you notice physiological cues like your eyes starting to involuntarily close or your head creaking back and forth, get into bed.

MAKE AN ACTION PLAN

Although many of these strategies may be used by themselves, most will need to be used in conjunction with others to address your insomnia effectively. Because of this, it'll be beneficial to come up with an action plan to address your insomnia.

After you've identified the sleep hygiene strategies you need to implement from the sidebar on page 36, you can then identify what your sleep disruptors are from "Increase Your Insight" on page 31. Next, add the corresponding items from each disruptor to your action plan.

On the next page you will find a sample action plan for an individual with all three sleep disruptors who was not following all of the sleep hygiene rules and has decided to start with stimulus control therapy.

Sample Plan:

PAGE #	STRATEGY NAME	DISRUPTOR ADDRESSED
44	Nix the Caffeine	Hygiene (Homeostat-Related)
54	Get Your Body Moving	Hygiene (Homeostat-Related)
65	Food Timing	Hygiene (Arousal-Related)
113	Keep It Cool	Hygiene (Arousal-Related)
25	Rhythm—You Can Feel It	Clock
27	Quit *Lying* to Yourself	Arousal
42	Savor Your Bed	Arousal
46	You're Getting Sleepy	Homeostat
56	Leave Napping to Babies	Homeostat
87	Are You Really Sleepy?	Homeostat

Kick That Smoking Habit

WHY IT WORKS

By now, we all know the negative and deadly impacts smoking can have on your health, but did you know that it can also impact your sleep? Because nicotine is a stimulant, it influences your brain, and subsequently your sleep, in much the same way caffeine does. Not only does it impair your ability to fall asleep, but it can also reduce your ability to produce rapid eye movement and slow-wave sleep, which are restorative to our health. In fact, research proves that smokers have about twice the risk of experiencing sleep problems overall and also experience increased daytime sleepiness. Although it is very challenging to quit, it will benefit you in many ways overall.

Unfortunately, during early stages of withdrawal from nicotine, you may experience a decrease in overall sleep quality, more frequent and longer awakenings, and even an increase in depressive symptoms. It is important for you to follow the other strategies in this book and remind yourself that it will get better with time.

Grab a Surfboard:

Many people have found that practicing meditation can help you "surf" your urges more effectively— that is, noticing and becoming aware of the urge, describing it with openness and curiosity, and watching it subside. This takes a lot of practice, but it works if you engage in it repeatedly over time.

Reconsider That Nightcap

WHY IT WORKS

Many people believe having a drink or two after dinner or before bedtime will help them sleep. This couldn't be further from the truth. Alcohol is a sedative. In early stages of consumption, alcohol sedates your prefrontal cortex—the part of our brain that controls our impulses and helps us think and plan. With time, alcohol starts to sedate other parts of our brain, effectively sedating you out of wakefulness. However, the brainwaves produced during sedation are not what we experience in natural sleep. In fact, when we are "sleeping" under the influence of alcohol, we experience frequent awakenings, which impairs our ability to receive restorative sleep. Because your brain is still sedated, however, you do not remember them, causing you to believe you slept well, which is why many people have trouble realizing the "hangover" they experience the next day is in part due to their poor sleep. Additionally, alcohol prevents us from experiencing rapid eye movement (REM) sleep, which has important consequences for memory integration and association.

HOW TO DO IT

Instead of having that glass of wine to unwind after a long day, consider engaging in other types of relaxation strategies. Experiment with a few to find one that works the best for you. Some suggestions include lighting candles/incense, drinking herbal tea, giving yourself a massage, or engaging in deep breathing exercises. Once you start getting adequate sleep, you may not even want that nightcap.

Get Your Body Moving

WHY IT WORKS

Ever noticed how well you sleep after getting exercise? Then you've experienced what we know from dozens of clinical trials—exercise can improve your sleep quality, help you fall asleep faster, and reduce how much sleep medication you may be inclined to use. In adults, exercise increases the total time you are asleep as well as your overall sleep efficiency. It improves sleep by increasing energy consumption, endorphin secretion, or body temperature in a way that facilitates sleep for recuperation of the body. It's also thought to work by reducing stress and increasing sleep drive by tiring you out.

Exercise and sleep have a bidirectional relationship—the better you sleep, the more energy you will have to exercise, and the better you will sleep again. Slowly establishing an exercise routine will improve your sleep with time.

HOW TO DO IT

Consider making small, realistic, and attainable
goals to increase your overall level of physical
activity throughout your day (e.g., ten minutes a day,
three days a week). Too busy to make it to the gym
or go for a long run? Try making micro changes
like parking further away than usual, or walking
or biking to where you need to be if you are able.
Experiment with taking small breaks throughout
your day to go for a short walk or stretch.

Leave Napping to Babies

WHY IT WORKS

From the moment we get out of bed, our body is building up sleep drive so that by the time we lay our head on our pillow again, we can easily fall asleep. However, when we take naps, our sleep drive gets deflated, and the longer we nap and/or are sedentary, the weaker our sleep drive will be.

This deflation causes us to have difficulty falling asleep, and also impedes our ability to receive the deeper, more restorative sleep our body needs to work optimally. This may be difficult to accept, as the less you sleep at night, the more prone you may be to nap during the day, but allowing yourself to take that nap will, unfortunately, make matters worse for you in the long run. So, it's better to leave the napping to babies until you can get your sleep back on track.

The next time you are tempted to take a nap, first assess whether you absolutely need to take a nap for safety reasons (e.g., you need to drive, operate heavy machinery, etc.). If that is the case, go ahead and nap for as long as you need to in order to keep yourself safe. But if you just want to take a nap because you feel fatigued, try taking a brief walk or engaging in some gentle stretching if your body will allow it. Remind yourself that delayed gratification is always more rewarding.

Dispelling the Sleeping Pill Myth

WHY IT WORKS

Sleeping pills (e.g., Ambien, Lunesta) impact us in much the same way alcohol does, by sedating our brain so that we think we are asleep. The brainwaves produced while asleep when taking these drugs are vastly different than those that are produced naturally. It is more akin to what it would look like if you were under anesthesia. You may think you are getting more sleep, but objectively, you are not. Without natural sleep, we risk detrimental health consequences, like memory loss, the ability to ward of illness or infection, and our overall longevity.

To make matters worse, sleeping pill use is also correlated to an increased risk for fatal car accidents, higher rates of heart disease and stroke, and increased risk of cancer. When you discontinue sleeping pills, you experience rebound insomnia, which can make it more likely that you start taking them again, leading to a never-ending cycle—all the more reason why treating your insomnia the natural way is better for you in the long run.

HOW TO DO IT

CBT-I is proven to be just as effective for those currently on sleep medications. Experiment with the other skills in this book to help you get a better hold on your symptoms. When you are ready, speak with your doctor about tapering off your medication. It can also be helpful to have a trained CBT-I therapist guide you through this process.

MARY'S SLEEP STORY

When Mary first began seeing me for treatment, she'd been experiencing insomnia for over ten months. With tears rolling down her cheeks, she told me she'd tried everything she could think of to get rid of her insomnia—from various prescription medications, herbs, and oils, to hypnosis, meditation, and tapping.

Through our conversations, she discovered that staying in bed when she was not sleeping was actually contributing to increasing levels of fragmented sleep and hyperarousal in the long term.

Based on her sleep diaries, we identified that a combination of sleep restriction, stimulus control, and relaxation methods would be most beneficial in addressing her symptoms.

Armed with coping statements and counter-arousal strategies, Mary trekked on with the plan we set in place, eventually increasing her time in bed to seven and a half hours within eight weeks. Her faith in her body's natural ability to produce sleep had finally been restored.

No Effort Required

WHY IT WORKS

If we start worrying that we need to exert effort to *try* to go to sleep, it leads to increased anxiety, which weakens our ability to produce sleep. Months to years of sleepless nights mean we might start taking sleeping pills, herbs, or substances, or making sure we have the latest device that promises to help us sleep. Continuing to engage in these "sleep effort" behaviors just perpetuates the problem. One of the best things we can do is to actually remind ourselves that *trying* hasn't worked so well for us in the past, so maybe it's better not to try and see what happens.

The next time you notice yourself thinking about which new sleep aid, device, or other non-evidence-based item you are going to use, take a step back and examine your thoughts. Are you starting to feel more anxious because you believe you won't be able to sleep without these things? Gently remind yourself that it's actually the anxiety you've developed around your sleep that's preventing you from sleeping. You can experiment with writing out phrases such as, "Sleep will come naturally if I don't try." If you catch yourself in bed *trying* to sleep, it just means you aren't ready for sleep yet, so get up and do something calming and relaxing, such as reading a book or listening to music (see "Plan for Not Sleeping" on page 146 for more suggestions) until you no longer need to try.

S.T.O.P. Your Stress

WHY IT WORKS

Our arousal system, also known as our fight-or-flight response, gets our body prepared to adequately respond to danger. When it's overactivated, it overrides our sleep-promoting system. After all, it wouldn't help us if we were sleepy when we needed to respond to a threat.

One of the biggest contributors to an overloaded arousal system is stress and anxiety. Many times, we don't notice how stressed we are until our head hits the pillow and our mind starts racing. Learning to better manage your anxiety during the day will help you take back control of your night. While "Schedule 'Worry' Time" on page 38 works to reduce arousal by actively scheduling a time every day to write down your worries, you can also take a more mindful approach. Take brief moments informally throughout your day to check in with your thoughts and notice them pass without writing them down, judging them, or trying to work through them.

Take brief moments to **S.T.O.P.** regularly through-out your day:

1. **S** = Stop what you are doing.
2. **T** = Take a few deep breaths.
3. **O** = Observe your thoughts. If you notice any tension or stress, don't judge it, just name the feeling to yourself. Remind yourself that your thoughts are just thoughts, not facts.
4. **P** = Proceed with anything that will help soothe you—like sipping on a cup of chamomile tea, talking to a trusted friend, etc.

Food Timing

WHY IT WORKS

Consuming a heavy meal too close to your bedtime may cause you to experience indigestion, constipation, heartburn, or even nausea, which can make you feel very uncomfortable and thus make it harder for you to fall asleep. Our bodies are made to digest food in an upright position. Lying down soon after consuming a heavy meal can cause you to experience indigestion as it encourages food to move back up, out of your stomach, and into your esophagus. Remaining upright for two to three hours after a large meal will lessen the risk of experiencing these uncomfortable symptoms. Individuals with gastro-esophageal reflux disease, irritable bowel syndrome, and inflammatory bowel diseases are even more prone to experience insomnia due to gastrointestinal issues. It's especially important for those with these conditions to avoid heavy meals and spicy or sugary trigger foods at least two to three hours before bedtime.

HOW TO DO IT

If you are prone to consuming your last meal right before bed, take a moment to examine your schedule and determine whether it is absolutely necessary for you to be eating so late. If work demands make it impossible to get around this, try to build in more opportunities for smaller meals earlier in your day to avoid feeling ravenous when you get home. You may want to consider engaging in some meal prep on your days off to make this easier.

Birds of a Feather Sleep Together

WHY IT WORKS

Our twenty-four-hour biological clock is controlled by a tiny structure in the middle of our brain called the suprachiasmatic nucleus (SCN). One responsibility of the SCN is to determine the level of wakefulness or sleepiness we feel throughout the day. But our clocks are not all the same—our genes are responsible for making us either more prone to sleep and wake up late ("night owls") or get up before dawn ("morning larks").

There were important evolutionary reasons for these differences—consider our ancestors who needed to be on night watch for danger. But due to the way our modern society has been established (especially with regards to work schedules), it is usually the owls, who account for about 30% of the population, who get the short end of the stick.

Determining your own chronotype will both help you distinguish between having a circadian rhythm disorder versus insomnia and will also help you determine your ideal bed and rise times.

HOW TO DO IT

There are questionnaires you can take online to determine your level of morningness versus eveningness (the Center for Environmental Therapeutics has an automated version on their website). Then, you can match up your bed and rise times closer to your biology. If you can't get around this because of work schedules or other factors and it is causing you severe distress, consider seeing a sleep specialist who can provide you with a specific plan—usually involving carefully timed exposure to light and the use of melatonin—to better address your symptoms.

No Pain, No Gain

WHY IT WORKS

The longer we linger in bed, the more fragmented our sleep becomes, and the less opportunity our body has to build up adenosine—the chemical responsible for our sleep drive. You may want to see "You're Getting Sleepy" on page 46 to help determine when you should be getting into bed. Instead, the old adage "no pain, no gain" applies here—we have to sacrifice one night of sleep to get better sleep the next night. If that's making you squirm, just know this is by far one of the most effective techniques to help get your sleep back on track.

1. Use a sleep diary (like the "CBT-i Coach" app or the one on page 22) to record your sleep for a one- to two-week period and determine your Average Total Sleep Time (ATST; calculated by adding the number of hours you slept each night and dividing by the total number of nights recorded).

2. Add thirty minutes to your ATST to determine your Time In Bed (TIB)—this will be the total amount of time you are allowed to be in bed every night. Don't ever give yourself less than five and a half hours of TIB unless told to do so by a sleep specialist.

3. Set a consistent rise and wake time based on your schedule, determined TIB, and chronotype. Stick to this for two weeks and continue to record your sleep. Go to bed when you are sleepy, but not before your earliest bedtime every night.

4. Calculate your sleep efficiency percentage after two weeks with this formula: (ATST / Average TIB) × 100.

5. Once your sleep efficiency is over 90%, you can increase the amount of time you spend in bed weekly by fifteen- to thirty-minute increments until you are no longer sleepy during the day (see "Assess Your Alertness" on page 126 for more information on how to determine your optimal amount of sleep).

INSOMNIA OR CIRCADIAN RHYTHM DISORDER?

We all have different chronotypes, or biological rhythms, that control the timing of our sleep. But some people have more definite morning or evening tendencies.

Individuals who are morning types can fall asleep as early as 8 p.m. and wake up around 3 or 4 a.m. Evening types will naturally fall asleep around 2 a.m. and wake up around 10 a.m. People who fall into these categories and don't know it may think they are experiencing an insomnia disorder. But they actually have a circadian rhythm disorder.

Those who are required to keep a schedule inconsistent with their biology may require treatment, especially if they experience sleepiness or insomnia plus its accompanying distress or impairment. While many of the sleep hygiene recommendations in this book will still be helpful, they will not properly address your symptoms. Reaching out to a sleep specialist in this case will be most beneficial.

Visual Imagery

WHY IT WORKS

Not being able to quiet down worries about work, family, friends, health, and so on is one of the most common reasons people give for being unable to fall asleep. When we experience these thoughts, our brain and body jump into fight-or-flight mode, making it very challenging for us to rest.

But if we are able to take up enough "cognitive space" with another mental activity, it is hard for our brain to simultaneously focus on our worries. One method researchers have found to help block out unwanted thoughts is imagery training.

HOW TO DO IT

1. About ten to fifteen minutes before you get in bed, select a situation you would like to imagine that you find interesting but also pleasant and relaxing.
2. Once in bed, close your eyes and spend five minutes imagining the scene you have chosen in as much detail as possible.

3. Ask yourself the following questions to make the scene vivid:
   a. What can you see around you?
   b. How are you feeling?
   c. What can you feel around you?
   d. Are you able to hear any sounds or voices?
   e. What is the general atmosphere like?
4. Keep imagining the situation until sleep overcomes you.
5. Try this out every night for one week. After that, keep track of how long it takes you to fall asleep. If you are able to fall asleep faster than before you tried it, keep engaging in this exercise.

Be a Paradox

WHY IT WORKS

We cannot voluntarily control our natural ability to produce sleep. Any attempt to "will" ourselves to sleep (usually in the form of lying completely still, shutting our eyes tight, and repeating to ourselves, "Fall asleep!") fails because we're prevented from feeling relaxed. We're creating too much performance anxiety. Think about what happens if you've ever been too anxious before a big gig or exam—you most likely didn't do so well. The same applies to our sleep. Knowing this, scientists decided to examine what happens if you do the exact opposite, i.e., try to not fall asleep. Will you actually then be able to sleep? It turns out, you will. If we are able to reduce our performance anxiety around sleep by diverting our attention, it reduces our level of anxiety and arousal thereby helping us fall asleep much faster.

For the next two weeks, when you get in bed and turn out the lights, try to stay awake for as long as possible by keeping your eyes open. Make sure your bed and bedroom are set up such that sleep will naturally come (i.e., block out noise and light and keep the temperature cool), but allow yourself to gently resist falling asleep. Don't engage in any active methods to prevent yourself from sleeping, such as reading, watching TV, or moving around. Keep in mind that this method is more helpful for those who have difficulty falling asleep.

Reduce Your Blues

WHY IT WORKS

As you may recall from a previous strategy, the structure in our brain responsible for the timing of our circadian system is called the suprachiasmatic nucleus (SCN). It resets our clock every day by sensing light signals, which are most sensitive to blue spectrum lights.

With the invention of lightbulbs, everything changed. We were no longer falling asleep a few hours after dusk because the light receptors in our eyes began communicating to our SCN that it was still "daylight." And with the advent of blue light emitting LED lights, which power our laptop screens, smartphones, and tablets, the problem grew worse. Studies now show that using these devices at night can delay the rise of melatonin (the hormone our body produces to promote sleep) by up to three hours, preventing us from falling asleep, and can even decrease the overall quality of our sleep and our level of alertness the next day.

HOW TO DO IT

While it's best to give your eyes a "lights out" two to three hours before bedtime by turning off all screens and devices, you might find this challenging. Almost all devices have built-in settings or apps available for download that allow you to reduce blue light. If you've grown accustomed to reading a book on a device, try going old-fashioned and switching back to the classic paper book. You can also purchase blue light reducing glasses as an alternative.

Keep It Quiet

WHY IT WORKS

This one might seem obvious, but the noisier our environment, the higher our chances will be of experiencing fragmented, lower-quality sleep and reduced total sleep time. Humans are able to perceive, evaluate, and even react to sounds while asleep. The degree to which noise can impact our sleep depends on what sleep stage we are in, the existing background noise level, and an individual's unique noise sensitivity. While we don't yet know exactly what can predict an individual's sensitivity to noise, we do know that certain groups are at higher risk for noise-induced sleep disturbance—older adults, children, shift workers, and especially those who have preexisting sleep disorders, such as insomnia.

HOW TO DO IT

Try experimenting with different methods to block
out noise from your bedroom, such as using earplugs, wearing headphones, installing blackout
shades (which reduce both light and noise), or using
a "white noise" machine. There are many apps available for download that can produce calming sounds
which may help you drown out more disruptive
noises. Many people have also grown accustomed
to falling asleep with the TV, and they find that
while it helps them fall asleep, they tend to wake up
in the middle of the night, usually because sounds
get louder during commercials. If you fall into this
category, try setting a timer on your TV so that it
automatically turns off after thirty to sixty minutes.

Let Those Muscles Relax

WHY IT WORKS

Anxiety and stress can activate our fight-or-flight response. When we experience chronic stress, our brain's ability to reduce this response is weakened over time. This leaves us at risk for experiencing physical pain, which can make it harder for us to fall asleep and stay asleep. Through a technique called progressive muscle relaxation (PMR), you can relieve the tension in your body by tensing and releasing different muscle groups one at a time.

HOW TO DO IT

Comfortably lie down on your back, ideally not on the bed. It may be helpful for you to practice PMR by starting at one end of your body and working your way to the other. Try starting with either your feet or your shoulders.

1. Close your eyes if you're comfortable doing so. Breathe in, and tense the first muscle group hard, but not to the point of pain, for five seconds.

2. Breathe out, and immediately relax the muscle group all at once.

3. Take a few deep breaths for ten to fifteen seconds before moving on to the next muscle group. During this time, pay attention to how the muscles feel when they are tense versus relaxed.

4. Repeat steps one through three with each muscle group.

5. When you are finished with all of the muscle groups, take the deepest breath you've taken in all day and let it out. When you are ready, bring your focus back to the present.

INSOMNIA DISORDER
VERSUS ANXIETY DISORDER

Individuals with insomnia often also experience anxiety. While the anxiety that insomniacs experience is usually centered around sleep, some individuals also have a coexisting anxiety disorder—most commonly Generalized Anxiety Disorder (GAD) or panic disorder. People often experience confusion around whether they have an anxiety disorder, an insomnia disorder, or both.

The key difference is that, in GAD, the individual is worrying about *many* topics, not just the fact that they can't sleep. Similarly, in panic disorder, the main focus of worry is on experiencing panic attacks.

We used to think that having an anxiety disorder caused you to develop insomnia, but we now know that the relationship is bidirectional—either one can cause the other. Taking proactive steps toward addressing your insomnia can either prevent these additional disorders from developing, or provide you with more rapid recovery of your existing anxiety symptoms.

You Are Not Broken

WHY IT WORKS

Everyone experiences the occasional sleepless night from time to time. But, when you continue to experience insomnia for months on end, it can be easy to start to lose hope and begin to think that normal sleep might not ever come again. While it is completely understandable if your mind has started to go here, the unfortunate consequence is that these thoughts can make you feel more anxious and stressed and cause you to unconsciously behave in ways that not only exacerbate your anxiety, but also reinforce your insomnia.

For example, you might be thinking, "I haven't slept in months. I'm probably never going to be able to sleep again. Something is seriously wrong with me," which causes you to feel anxious. When you get into bed at night, these thoughts continue to spiral through your mind and you become too physiologically aroused to fall asleep. You then decide, "Let me take a sleep aid to at least get some reprieve." And you do get a little more "sleep" that night (although you are really just sedated). Your thought the next day is, "I tried my hardest to sleep but nothing worked except that pill so I must need it to sleep." The cycle continues the next night, further reinforcing an underlying belief that "I can't sleep naturally, so I must be *broken*."

You can break this chain, however, by learning how to work through these thoughts. This will decrease your anxiety, allow you to break free from unhealthy habits, and finally provide natural sleep.

HOW TO DO IT

1. Pay attention to cues you are feeling anxious or distressed (e.g., shallow breathing, accelerated heart rate, shaking, sweating, feeling on edge, ruminating, and restlessness).

2. Every time you notice anxiety, take a moment to write down what you are thinking.

3. Examine the evidence for and against your thoughts and generate alternative ways of thinking. Do this every day until you no longer believe the anxiety-provoking thought. Example:

THOUGHT	FEELING	EVIDENCE FOR THOUGHT	EVIDENCE AGAINST THOUGHT	ALTERNATIVE THOUGHT
I will never be able to sleep again.	Anxiety	I didn't sleep at all last night.	I was able to sleep a few hours the previous night. I've had many more nights of normal sleep than no sleep.	Although it was stressful to not sleep last night, I know I can sleep again in the future.

Are You Really Sleepy?

WHY IT WORKS

Your experience with insomnia has probably set you up to become acutely aware of how *tired* you feel throughout the day, but not how *sleepy* you feel. This might sound like semantics, but there's a big difference. The former is associated with your level of fatigue, which can be caused by many factors other than just sleep, and the latter is associated with how ready your body is in that moment to fall asleep quickly and with ease.

Not knowing your sleepy cues can mean you decide to get in bed when you are not really ready for sleep. This sets you up for a pattern of getting into bed and not being able to fall asleep, perpetuating your insomnia. If you learn to pay attention to your sleepy cues, you can break this cycle.

Here are some cues to look out for to determine whether you are actually sleepy:

1. Eyes involuntarily closing
2. Head creaking back and forth
3. Involuntary dozing
4. Zoning out (e.g., if you are watching TV or reading something, notice if you keep having to reread passages or rewind the show)
5. Feeling colder

If you do not notice any of these signs, remind yourself that you are not ready for sleep yet—continue to stay out of bed and engage in relaxing and non-stimulating activities (e.g., reading a book, listening to music, writing, deep breathing) until you notice one or more of these cues.

Write It Out

WHY IT WORKS

While there may be various reasons why negative thoughts flood your mind as soon as your head hits the pillow, one hypothesis researchers have posed is that bedtime is the first quiet moment you might have to finally reflect about your day or plan for the future.

Researchers have found engaging in expressive writing before bed can reduce levels of cognitive arousal and reduce the time it takes you to fall asleep. Writing about your emotions can assist you in organizing and processing distressing events and letting them go or letting them be, thereby freeing up your mind to help you sleep. Writing down your thoughts and feelings can also increase your general health and well-being.

Before getting into bed, spend twenty minutes writing down any thoughts, concerns, or worries. You can record yourself speaking if writing is not possible or too challenging. Try to be as open and honest as you can, without worrying about spelling or grammar.

Write Now:

Try this out every day for one week. Here are some prompts to get you started:

- How did your day start and end? Did you experience anything stressful, challenging, or positive?

- What's been worrying you? When did these worries start? How do you think they'll impact you in the future?

- Is there something you've been thinking about several times in the last few days? Write how you feel about it.

Just Breathe

WHY IT WORKS

To ensure our survival, our body has come up
with quick ways to prepare us for danger. When
we perceive a threat, our sympathetic nervous
system (the fight-or-flight response) gets activated.
That triggers a release of hormones, starting with
adrenaline, which leads to a cascade of physiological responses such as increased heart rate, blood
flow, metabolic rate, and core body temperature,
making it very challenging for us to fall asleep.
Chronic stress weakens our ability to "turn off"
this response in the absence of danger, leaving our
bodies in a state of constant physiological arousal
that can lead to a host of health problems, including insomnia. Practicing diaphragmatic breathing
(or belly breathing) once or twice a day can actually reduce these effects and help us achieve
better sleep.

1. Find a comfortable posture, either sitting upright in a chair or lying on the floor. Relax your shoulders.
2. Place one hand on your chest and the other hand on your stomach.
3. Take a deep breath in through your nose for about two to three seconds, trying to make the hand on your belly rise while the hand on your chest remains still.
4. Slowly and with control exhale through your mouth for about four to five seconds, as the hand on your belly falls.
5. Repeat at least ten times or until you notice yourself feeling more relaxed.

Fighting the Fight-or-Flight Response

WHY IT WORKS

Chronic stress has been strongly linked to insomnia. Even positive situations such as getting married or purchasing a home can cause us stress. External causes like work and relationship difficulties and internal causes like negative self-talk and perfectionism all cause stress.

Whatever the cause, our body reacts in the same way—by activating our fight-or-flight response. In doing so, the body stays on high alert, preventing us from falling asleep.

More and more of us face chronic high levels of stress, especially internal pressures, which keeps this system constantly activated and contributes to a multitude of health issues, such as high blood pressure and weight gain. Fortunately, chronic stress can be managed with lifestyle and behavior changes, which can, in turn, improve sleep.

HOW TO DO IT

1. Write down your internal, external, positive, and negative sources of stress.

2. Identify any steps you can take to better manage some of these stressors. Are there tasks you can cut back on? Can you ask for assistance from friends or family?

3. For the stressors you either don't have control over or know will not immediately change, working toward acceptance can be very beneficial. It is often the way we *think* about situations, rather than the actual situation itself, that causes us to experience stress. You may find "Challenge Unhelpful Thoughts" on page 157, "Practice Mindfulness" on page 148, and "Get Off the Thought Train" on page 174 particularly helpful with this.

SLEEP AND WEIGHT GAIN

It is well established that sleeping only four to five hours per night is associated with weight gain. There are several reasons for this. First, we wind up with decreased concentrations of leptin, the hormone that signals to your brain that you are full. We also get increased concentrations of ghrelin, the hormone that triggers hunger sensations, and endocannabinoids, which stimulate appetite.

We additionally experience reduced activity in the prefrontal cortex of our brain, which is responsible for controlling our decisions, as well as increased activity in the deep brain structures that drive motivation and desire, contributing to poorer food choices.

The good news is taking active steps toward addressing your insomnia and getting better sleep can help reverse these effects and keep you happier and healthier overall.

If at First You Don't Succeed

WHY IT WORKS

It took many weeks, months, or even years for your insomnia to get to the point that it has. We can't expect that it will only take a matter of days to recover. One of the primary reasons people fail to effectively address their insomnia is because they give up too quickly. While it can be very challenging to implement some of these strategies, it is important for you to understand what is getting in the way of you being successful enough to actually start seeing results. Then, you can come up with solutions to get yourself back on track.

HOW TO DO IT

Get to the root of what's blocking your progress by following these steps:

1. Write down which strategies you have tried so far and how long you tried them.

2. Star any strategies you used for less than a week or have only used intermittently (when not instructed to).

3. Star any strategies you didn't follow completely.

4. Go through each strategy you starred and identify why it was difficult for you to follow. Were you expecting to see change after a few days, and when you didn't, you gave up? Did you set an unrealistic sleep schedule based on your chronotype?

5. Notice any patterns or common themes, and start to identify strategies to counteract each. Turn the page to learn how to do just that! After all, what good are identifying your problems if we don't come up with some solutions?

Create Solutions

WHY IT WORKS

New behaviors are often not as motivating as existing ones that have been previously rewarded. For example, why get up earlier in order to stick to a schedule to improve your sleep in the long run if you already know that letting yourself sleep in will be immediately rewarding?

In order to be successful in conquering your insomnia, you need to become your own motivator. First, identify what might be getting in the way of your success, and then identify solutions to overcome these barriers.

HOW TO DO IT

1. Identify your barriers toward change. That's the exercise you completed in the previous strategy, "If at First You Don't Succeed." If you skipped that one, go back and take a look at it now.

2. On a sheet of paper, create three columns—one for the strategy you are or have been trying, one for

your barriers toward implementing the strategy, and one for solutions.

3. Fill out the first two columns by listing the strategy in the leftmost column and the barriers for that strategy in the column next to it.

4. Now start identifying possible solutions for each barrier in the right column. Example:

STRATEGY	BARRIER	SOLUTION
Get out of bed if you haven't fallen asleep within twenty minutes.	*My wife will feel abandoned if I keep getting out of bed.*	*My wife knows how much my insomnia is impacting me and wants me to get better.* *We can schedule quality time with each other on the weekends.*

5. Now that you have identified solutions, put them into practice. Keep this worksheet and review it daily as a reminder to keep yourself motivated.

Give Yourself Permission to "Be"

WHY IT WORKS

Sometimes life gets so hectic that scheduling yourself for every waking hour of the day seems like it can't be helped. But, constantly operating in this "doing" mode—where your focus is always on getting things done—prevents you from being present with your current experiences. This can make it harder for us to recognize and release any tension we might be carrying from our day, which then impacts our sleep. Providing yourself moments to practice operating out of "being" mode instead, allows you to more easily let things go or be.

HOW TO DO IT

For the next two weeks, provide yourself with more opportunities to be with your present experience. Do so with kindness and without any goal or judgment. Here are some examples:

- During your next meal, try not to engage in any other activities besides eating. Spend time really focusing on what your food looks, smells, feels, and tastes like. Describe these sensations to yourself.

- When walking from one point to another, like from your office to the conference room, try to focus on what it feels like to be walking without paying attention to other things. Notice one foot lifting off the floor and then being placed on the floor again, then notice the opposite foot. If your mind gets distracted with something else, just bring it back to the sensation of walking.

- For two to three minutes, take a look around you and describe what you notice and what you feel in your body.

Cognitive Distraction

WHY IT WORKS

Certain activities can help distract you from anxiety-provoking thoughts that make it hard to sleep. Think about what happens when you're watching your favorite TV show or having a meaningful conversation. While your worries may still be present somewhere in the back of your mind, it's harder for you to actively focus on them if you are attuned to the present moment or engaged in something else. Research shows that cognitive distraction techniques, such as the one presented next, reduces the amount of time it takes you to fall asleep for this reason.

HOW TO DO IT

1. Pick a novel you would like to read or listen to.
2. Spend about thirty minutes reading or listening to it.
3. Immediately after you stop reading/listening, get into bed and try to imagine what happens next in

the story, making it as real as possible. What are the characters in the story saying or doing? Where are they located?

4. Continue to engage in this until sleep takes over.

Engage in this practice every night for one week. Think about how long it takes you to fall asleep. If you imagine a scenario that was too exciting, try a different book that is not as stimulating instead.

Note: Remember to keep recording your sleep before you start using these strategies and continue to record while you use them (using the sleep diary on page 22), so you can determine whether they increase your total sleep time.

Are Medications the Culprit?

WHY IT WORKS

Our sleep structure is cyclical and is composed of non-rapid eye movement (NREM; which has several stages) sleep and rapid eye movement (REM) sleep.

Unfortunately, many commonly used medications used to treat pain, depression, and some cardiac and pulmonary problems, impact the quality and architecture of our sleep. Opioids, for example, decrease both slow-wave sleep, which is the most restorative, and REM sleep. Abruptly discontinuing these medications can cause you to experience what is called REM rebound—your body's way of making up for all of the REM you were losing while it was being suppressed. REM rebound may cause you to experience more intense or vivid dreams, and even nightmares, which may be bothersome and can contribute to insomnia. Nonsteroidal anti-inflammatory drugs (NSAIDS), such as aspirin, can also decrease slow-wave sleep, causing you to experiencing more lighter stages of sleep, in which you are more prone to awakenings.

HOW TO DO IT

If you are currently taking any medications, it will be important for you to discuss with your prescriber if and how any of these medications may be impacting your sleep. Explore whether any of your medications can be changed or augmented to improve your sleep. If you're discontinuing any medications, talk to your provider about any potential withdrawal effects so that they can better support you. This may also be the time to seek additional support from a behavioral sleep medicine specialist.

SLEEP STAGES

Your brain cycles through five stages of sleep every ninety minutes: non-rapid eye movement sleep (NREM: Stages 1 to 4) and rapid eye movement sleep (REM).

NREM Stage 1 is the lightest stage of sleep. During NREM Stage 2, your brain waves slow down and increase in frequency. NREM Stages 3 and 4 are when the most restoration to your body occurs.

Most of your dreaming and memory consolidation happens during REM sleep.

The less you sleep, the more your body will make up Stages 3 and 4. We all have less memory for Stages 3 and 4 of sleep, and insomniacs in particular perceive Stages 1 and 2 as being awake (even though objective tests of sleep prove the opposite). People with insomnia then believe they haven't slept at all, when that is not the case.

This is why it is so helpful to challenge your thinking around sleep.

Rumination Causes Rumination

WHY IT WORKS

A common problem people with insomnia face is rumination—the constant rehashing of a thought or concern in your mind. Over time, ruminating can become habitual—certain feelings, locations, or situations can cause you to ruminate automatically. Every time you ruminate, your fight-or-flight response gets activated, which prevents you from falling asleep. Luckily, the following is a well-researched method proven to help you reduce your rumination.

HOW TO DO IT

1. Build awareness. Every time you think you may be ruminating, continue what you are doing for about

two more minutes, then ask yourself the following questions:

   a. Did you learn anything new?

   b. Are you any closer to a solution?

   c. Do you feel any better?

2. If you answered no to any of the above questions, you are ruminating.

3. Identify if there are any triggers. Keep a daily log of the circumstances that occur right before you begin ruminating. This could include the time of day, location, and whether it's occurring during another routine activity, such as driving home, or a feeling, such as being fatigued.

4. Now that you have identified your triggers, alter or remove them if possible. For example, if you ruminate when you are tired, engage in a thought record (see "You Are Not Broken" on page 84) or engage in some light stretching.

5. Repeat this process whenever you catch yourself ruminating until you no longer notice the tendency to ruminate. This will take practice, so be patient and kind to yourself.

Food for Sleep

WHY IT WORKS

What we eat, how much we eat, and when we eat can all impact our sleep. Spicy, acidic, and high-fat foods all stimulate acid production, making you more prone to heartburn, which can cause discomfort, making it difficult to fall or stay asleep. Foods with refined carbohydrates or too much sugar lead to a spike in blood sugar and insulin levels, which quickly deplete. This leaves you more likely to feel hungry very soon after eating, which can cause you to wake up.

On the other hand, some foods can actually help promote sleep—those high in the amino acid tryptophan, found in foods containing protein. When we consume foods with tryptophan, it triggers serotonin (responsible for regulating positive mood, sleep, appetite, digestion, and memory) and melatonin (the hormone that controls our sleep drive) production, which help us both fall asleep and stay asleep.

- Limit spicy, acidic, high-fat, and sugary foods, especially three to four hours before bedtime.
- Try to incorporate foods containing tryptophan into your diet. Examples include:
  - Nuts and seeds
  - Legumes
  - Fruits
  - Vegetables
  - Grains
  - Dairy products
  - Poultry
  - Seafood
- Every day for two weeks, keep track of what, when, and how much you consume in conjunction with your sleep (see "Keep a Sleep Diary" on page 21 for instructions on how to record sleep).

But First, Sleep

WHY IT WORKS

Millions of people are constantly engaging in some form of social media use. But it can be too stimulating, preventing you from being able to receive adequate sleep. You may not realize just how much time you are spending at night posting updates or scrolling through your feed, which cuts into your total sleep time. Additionally, if you engage in a heated discussion, this may lead you to become emotionally, cognitively, and physiologically aroused. Plus, smartphones, laptops, tablets, and even the TV all use LED screens. The light emitted from these devices tricks our brain into thinking it is still daytime. In fact, one recent study found that young adults who engage in social media use with higher volume and frequency had greater odds of sleep disturbance, and those who obsessively checked their social media (more than seven to eight times per day, even if only briefly) had even greater disturbance.

Here are some methods to decrease social media use:

- Download an app to tell you how much time you're spending online (e.g., Moment).

- If you're prone to obsessively checking, see if you can go one week not checking for at least fifteen minutes at a time. Then, slowly increase the increments.

- Set specific hours for being tech-free, especially before bed.

- Use an alarm clock and/or a wristwatch. This will decrease the number of times you look at your phone.

Keep It Cool

WHY IT WORKS

Your twenty-four-hour biological clock, which among many things controls when you are awake or asleep is controlled by a tiny structure whose name you may recall from earlier in this book: the suprachiasmatic nucleus (SCN). During daylight hours, the SCN sends many signals to your brain and body that it is time to be awake and alert. At nighttime, these signals drop, which alert your brain that it is time to sleep.

One of the signals that drops at nighttime is your core body temperature. During your typical bedtime (which varies from person to person based on their unique biology), your SCN coordinates a drop in your body temperature that reaches its lowest point approximately two hours later. Your body temperature then slowly rises throughout the early morning, which helps alert your brain that it is time to wake up. If your body temperature is too high before bedtime or increases too much while you are asleep, however, it will be harder to fall asleep and stay asleep.

HOW TO DO IT

1. Keep your bedroom temperature cool. An ideal temperature is in the mid-sixty-degree Fahrenheit range. If you get too cold in the middle of the night, use comforters or blankets to keep yourself warm.

2. Wear breathable clothing and use breathable bedding such as cotton or linen.

3. Opt for a firmer mattress or avoid mattresses that tend to conform to the body, like memory foam or latex, as these can trap heat.

Mattress Matters

WHY IT WORKS

When you lie down for an extended period, the weight of your body reduces blood flow in the area you're lying on, depriving your skin of oxygen and nutrients, and causing your pain sensors to send a message to your brain to roll over. If your mattress is uncomfortable, you'll do this repeatedly, which can lead to fragmented sleep. While changing your mattress might be a necessary component in addressing your insomnia, it's not a sufficient way to treat your insomnia on its own. You will also need to implement many of the other strategies in this book for lasting relief.

HOW TO DO IT

Ask yourself the following questions about your mattress:

* Is it uncomfortable and/or causing your pain to worsen?

- Is it sagging?

- Is your spine not aligned when you lie down? For back or stomach sleepers, your spine's natural S curve should be evident. For side sleepers, your spine should be straight from neck to bottom—so if you can slide a hand in the gap between body and mattress, it's not aligned.

- Are any allergy or asthma symptoms worsening without another identifiable culprit?

If you answered yes to any of these, it might be time to purchase a new mattress.

CHRONIC PAIN AND INSOMNIA

Individuals with chronic pain often experience disturbed sleep. Numerous awakenings due to pain and difficulty getting comfortable in bed cause fragmented nighttime sleep, which causes decreased pain tolerance, increased pain, and decreased growth hormone secretion. This leads to a vicious cycle of not getting the sleep you need because you are in pain, while also not being able to recover from your pain because you can't sleep.

Evidence from numerous studies prove that CBT-I works as well in those with chronic pain as it does in those who are pain-free. There is also evidence that it can even lessen the intensity of pain, as the metabolite for growth hormone increases post-treatment.

If you are like the millions of other Americans who suffer from a chronic pain condition and insomnia, know that you are not alone, and that giving some of these strategies a try can also be beneficial to you.

Try a Body Scan

WHY IT WORKS

Many of us carry aches, pains, and tension in our bodies, often without even realizing it. It can be easy to get wrapped up in thoughts about other things, such as how our day went or worries about the future, and not notice what we feel in our body. Without being aware of how uncomfortable we may feel, when we lie in bed at night we might find ourselves awake without really understanding why.

The first step in trying to ease our discomfort or pain is by noticing it when it first begins. Practicing a mindful meditation called the body scan can actually help us relate differently to our pain, allowing us to either release it or let it be, which helps us fall asleep. There have been several body scan meditations developed for use at bedtime.

1. When it is time for you to sleep, get in bed and close your eyes.

2. Pay attention to the different areas of your body, one by one. Simply feel what is there to feel, without judgment. Allow yourself to drift off if sleep overcomes you.

3. As you move through the different areas of the body, you may notice temperature, pressure, tingling, tension, touch, or no sensation at all. If you notice any areas of tension, you can imagine yourself breathing into that area to release it.

4. Spend one to two minutes in each area. Start with the feet, then move up the body, finishing by opening awareness to the entire body.

Tip:

You can find a free audio recording of a "Body Scan for Sleep" on the UCLA Mindful Awareness Research Center website.

Light It Up

WHY IT WORKS

We all work on a twenty-four-hour clock called the circadian rhythm. This clock determines when we want to be awake or asleep. In the absence of any exposure to light, our body clock naturally runs longer than a twenty-four-hour day. Because of this, our body uses cues from the environment to help reset our clock every day.

One of the main sources we use for this is sunlight. Being exposed to sunlight in the morning causes production of melatonin—the hormone responsible for alerting your brain that it is time for sleep—to occur earlier in the evening, allowing you to sleep easier at night.

The problem is, many of us are increasingly prone to staying indoors most of the day. It's important for those who work indoors to get outside periodically when possible.

HOW TO DO IT

If you primarily work indoors, try the following to increase your sunlight exposure during the day:

- Take a ten- to fifteen-minute walk outside before you go to work or during one of your breaks. Even if it is a cloudy day, you will still receive the benefits. If possible, don't wear sunglasses during this time as your brain will receive more light signals.

- If for some reason it is impossible for you to get outside, there are full-spectrum lightboxes you can purchase online that can also help.

Engage in either of these practices on a daily basis and notice if your sleep improves.

Understanding Fatigue

WHY IT WORKS

Not being able to obtain sufficient sleep causes us to feel tired during the day. Knowing this, our mind tends to then focus throughout the day on just how tired we feel. This causes you to experience increased anxiety about your lack of sleep, which, in turn, leads you to become too aroused to be able to obtain sufficient sleep at night.

There are often other factors besides lack of sleep that can cause us to experience daytime fatigue. However, when we are preoccupied with our sleep, we tend to not pay attention to these reasons. Being able to recognize other reasons for feeling tired can help you decrease your anxiety surrounding the impacts of poor sleep.

The next time you notice yourself worrying about how tired you feel because of your lack of sleep, investigate whether you are also experiencing any of these:

- Dehydration
- Boredom
- Caffeine crash
- Low, irritable, or tense mood
- Stress
- Pain
- Anxiety
- Being sedentary all day

- Being very physically active
- Eye strain
- Constipation
- Anemia
- Infections
- Hypothyroidism
- Can you think of others?

Were there any that applied to you? If so, take actionable steps to address these other causes. Dehydrated? Drink more water throughout the day. Stressed? Try one of the many stress reduction methods listed throughout this book. Remind yourself that focusing on how bad you feel is most likely not actually making you feel better.

Bathe Yourself to Sleep

WHY IT WORKS

As you may recall, your circadian rhythm controls many biological functions including your core body temperature. Your body temperature fluctuates throughout the day, and at night, it drops and cools, signaling to your brain that it is time for sleep.

Taking a warm shower or bath at night bolsters this thermoregulation process. Your body temperature rises due to the water, then falls when you are out of it. This rapid cooldown of body temperature allows you to fall asleep faster. Research studies have also proven that taking a warm bath or shower before bedtime facilitates earlier sleep onset. In addition to dropping your body temperature, showering or bathing can also bolster relaxation—it helps your muscles relax, allows you to disconnect for a bit, and can literally eliminate the toxins/allergens that accumulated on you that day. All of this reduces your level of arousal and increases your chances of sleeping better.

HOW TO DO IT

Sixty to ninety minutes before your scheduled bedtime, take a warm shower or bath. Ensure the temperature is not too cold or too hot, which will make you more alert. You can also try incorporating some essential oils like lavender into your routine or lighting some candles. As you bathe, try to focus on any pleasant sensations you notice, and every time your mind drifts off to your worries, gently bring yourself back to where you are.

Assess Your Alertness

WHY IT WORKS

Everyone's unique biology will determine the amount of sleep they need. For the vast majority of people, obtaining seven to eight hours of sleep per night is sufficient.

It will be helpful for you to assess approximately how much sleep you require to feel alert and optimally functional throughout your day. This strategy will be most useful if used in conjunction with the sleep restriction strategy (see "No Pain, No Gain" on page 69), as you can use it to gauge whether you need additional time in bed and determine your optimal amount of nightly sleep.

HOW TO DO IT

1. Follow the rules for sleep restriction on page 70 of this book.
2. After reaching a sleep efficiency greater than or equal to 90% for one week, ask yourself the

following questions about how you felt on average during the previous week:

a. Did you feel tired or drowsy most of the time?
b. Did you take naps or doze off more than once or twice?
c. Are you satisfied with the quantity of your sleep overall?

3. If you answered yes to question (a) or (b) or no to question (c), add fifteen to thirty minutes to your time in bed and continue to record your sleep. Continue these steps until you reach 85% to 90% sleep efficiency.

4. When you achieve 85% to 90% sleep efficiency and you answer no to questions (a) and (b) and yes to question (c), you have determined your optimal time in bed.

SLEEP ACROSS OUR LIFESPAN

Our sleep changes as we age. Prior to birth, human infants spend much of their time in the womb asleep. It is not until the final trimester that we see some signs of real wakefulness (for about two to three hours per day). While newborns require up to seventeen hours of sleep per day, their sleep needs gradually decline. Infants and young children sleep for short bouts throughout the day and night with numerous awakenings. By the age of four or five, children usually sleep through the night with only one daytime nap.

The circadian rhythm of young children also runs on an earlier schedule, causing them to fall asleep and wake up earlier. By puberty and during adolescence, the rhythm shifts to a very late schedule, but gets earlier again by middle-age and even earlier by late adulthood.

As we age, we are also less able to produce deep sleep, and our sleep becomes more fragmented. However, it is important to note that older adults actually need just as much sleep as younger adults.

A Lightbulb Moment

WHY IT WORKS

The light spectrum our eyes can perceive runs from shorter wavelengths (cooler violets and blues) to longer wavelengths (warmer yellows and reds). Sunlight produces a blend of all of these colors. When the sun sets, it signals to our brain that it is time for sleep by releasing melatonin. However, the light emitted from electric lightbulbs can trick our brain into thinking it is still daytime, delaying the release of melatonin, which prevents us from falling asleep. The light receptors in our eye, which communicate that it is still daytime to our brain, are most sensitive to short wavelength light within the blue spectrum. Because of this, light within the blue spectrum will impact our brain significantly more than light in the warmer spectrum.

Consider changing the lightbulbs in your home to those in the warmer color temperature range (yellowish-white through red). Color temperature is measured in Kelvin (K). Bulbs that are 2800 K or lower will produce warmer lighting. While LED bulbs used to only be produced in the cooler, blue temperature, you are now able to purchase them in warmer tones. Try to also reduce the lighting in your home at night—especially in the two to three hours before bedtime—by either installing a dimmer or keeping only a few lights on. Remember to also reduce the blue light emitted from your devices (see "Reduce Your Blues" on page 77 for more information).

Hydrate

WHY IT WORKS

Your overall fluid intake and timing can impact
your sleep. Dehydration can cause you to feel tired,
irritable, lethargic, and more prone to headaches and
muscle cramps (among other symptoms). Coupled
with lack of sleep, this can further increase your
anxiety about not sleeping and make it difficult
to fall asleep again at night. Not drinking enough
water during the day also makes you more prone
to experiencing nocturnal leg cramps and snoring
(because your mouth and nasal passages are dry).
If you save most or even all of your fluid intake for
night, you will be more prone to frequent awakenings due to a need to urinate. All-in-all, paying
attention to how much liquid you are consuming and
when will assist you in improving your sleep.

- Drink plenty of non-caffeinated fluids regularly throughout the day (especially earlier in the day). Water is best, as your body depends on it in order to survive.

    ◦ Aim for about 2.5 to 3.5 liters per day, depending on your gender (males typically require more than females), how active you are, the environment—the hotter it is, the more water you will need—and any health conditions.

- Reduce your fluid intake about two hours before bedtime (some water is fine, just focus on getting most of your fluid intake earlier in the day).

- Avoid alcohol in the few hours before bedtime and caffeine after lunch, as they will leave you dehydrated and also disrupt your sleep.

Partnering with Insomnia

WHY IT WORKS

Sleeping next to a partner can feel wonderful—*sometimes*. Other times it can wreak havoc on your sleep, especially if you are experiencing insomnia. Sleeping next to someone can cause a rise in your body temperature, which may alert your brain to wake up. Moreover, your bed partner's habits or behaviors, such as movements throughout the night, different sleep schedules, use of technology, or noises from snoring, may cause you to wake up. And, if this is a new partner, the novelty of the situation or being in an unfamiliar environment may cause you to experience increased anxiety, which might also impact your sleep.

If you think this may be a contributing factor, open communication and problem-solving can help.

Set aside some time to problem-solve with your partner. Here is a general guideline:

1. Schedule a time to talk well before bedtime and ideally when you are both calm and not distracted by other things.

2. Identify together what you both think some of the problems are with your sleeping arrangement. Write them down.

3. Make a list of as many potential solutions as you can think of. Perhaps you need a larger bed, separate blankets, treatment for sleep apnea if your partner snores, or earplugs.

4. Narrow down the possibilities by discussing the feasibility of each solution.

5. Finalize your plan and discuss what might get in the way of you both being able to follow through.

Morning Joy

WHY IT WORKS

Our body depends on a consistent rise time to reset our twenty-four-hour biological clock, or circadian rhythm, every morning. Waking up at different times every day can cause our body to get confused and think we have traveled to a different time zone. For example, let's say you allow yourself to sleep in three hours longer than usual on a Sunday. That night, you will have just as much trouble falling asleep as you would have if you had just traveled from the west coast to the east coast. Not only will your circadian rhythm delay the release of sleep signals to your brain, but you will also not have built up enough sleep drive. That'll make it difficult for you to fall asleep at your usual bedtime and harder to wake up the next morning.

HOW TO DO IT

1. Write down several ideas that will help you get up at a consistent time every day.

   a. Examples: treat yourself to a special breakfast or your favorite coffee, get in the shower as soon as you wake up, or schedule time to hangout or workout with a friend.

2. Try each one. Make notes on whether it helped motivate you to get out of bed.

3. Make the most motivating strategy a consistent part of your morning routine.

4. If all else fails, remind yourself that morning sleep is light, low-quality sleep anyway; it is better to get up so you can sleep better the next night.

Assess Your Apnea Risk

WHY IT WORKS

While insomnia is distressing and should not be ignored, if you have obstructive sleep apnea (OSA), that needs to be addressed first. OSA is a serious sleep disorder that causes your breathing to repeatedly start and stop while you're asleep. Not treating apnea can lead to consequences including increased mortality, stroke, depression, cardiac disease, high blood pressure, obesity, and type 2 diabetes, among others.

Treating insomnia without treating apnea first is not only unsafe, but ineffective. Once your apnea is under control (at a minimum of 75% of nights), you can address your insomnia.

Are you at risk for OSA?

1. Do you snore loudly? You may want to ask for input from your bed partner or any roommates to help determine this.

2. Do you often feel sleepy during the day? Do you often fall asleep when talking to someone or watching TV?

3. Has anyone seen you stop breathing or choke/gasp while you are asleep?

4. Do you have high blood pressure?

5. Is your body mass index more than 35 kg/m^2? The Mayo Clinic's website has a BMI calculator you can use to find out.

6. Are you older than 50?

7. Is your neck size larger than 17 inches if you are male and 16 inches if you are female?

8. Are you a male?

If you answered yes to three or more questions, see your physician for an evaluation of OSA.

WHEN TO SEEK HELP

If in reading this book you recognize the presence of another sleep disorder or an additional mental health condition, like depression or anxiety, it might be time for you to seek additional help.

The strategies in this book are not meant to be used for individuals with untreated sleep apnea or a circadian rhythm disorder. Sleep apnea can lead to many health problems if left untreated. It is very important that you seek medical attention from a sleep specialist immediately if you think you may have these conditions.

Although many of the strategies in this book should provide you with relief from your insomnia symptoms, it can also be helpful to reach out to a trained professional, such as a mental health provider with a specialty in insomnia or behavioral sleep medicine. A specialist can offer you support and guide you through any difficulties you might experience with implementation.

Create a Sleep Sanctuary

WHY IT WORKS

Some environments or situations naturally produce more feelings of relaxation than others—think of lounging at the beach versus sitting in hours of traffic. But, if we have enough negative experiences during a situation or location over time, our brain becomes conditioned to experience that same place we used to find relaxing as a source of stress and anxiety. Imagine if every time you went to the beach, you got into a horrible fight with a loved one. The same thing can happen to our bed and bedroom over time. Too many negative or arousing experiences can cause us to associate the bedroom with stress instead of sleep. Fortunately, we can counteract these effects by creating an environment more conducive to rest and relaxation.

- Keep your bedroom cool, dark, and quiet. See "Keep It Quiet" on page 79, "Keep it Cool" on page 113, and "Keep It Dark" on page 191 for tips.

- Consider making the bedroom a device-free zone. If leaving your phone outside the room causes you stress, at least place it somewhere where it can't easily be reached from your bed.

- Move any work stations out of the bedroom. If this is not possible, try creating some sort of visual separation between your bed and your work area by experimenting with moving furniture or using room dividers.

- Reduce clutter and keep things clean and tidy.

- Add in a few key items that spark joy and/or relaxation, like your favorite art piece, photos, or memorabilia.

- Try to avoid having intense conversations in your bedroom and remember to get out of your bed and bedroom if you can't fall asleep.

Multitask Your Way to Sleep

WHY IT WORKS

Contrary to popular belief, our brains are incapable of focusing on two tasks at once. Think of texting while driving—it might seem like you're able to do it, but your brain is really just shifting its focus very rapidly back and forth, causing us to be less efficient at both tasks (and, sadly, creating more accidents). While there are many detrimental impacts of multi-tasking, you can use it to your advantage at bedtime.

Although there are different methods you can use to distract yourself, one that many have found to be effective is through repeating a single word or engaging in challenging mental arithmetic. These tasks take up so much space in the articulatory loop in your brain that you are unable to focus on those other unwanted thoughts, thereby quieting your mind, reducing your arousal, and allowing you to drift off.

HOW TO DO IT

If you are bothered by unwanted thoughts in the beginning, middle, or end of your sleep period, try either of the following:

- Mentally repeat the word "the" to yourself in a non-regular manner (try different tones, inflections, or speeds to distract your mind) continuously until you fall asleep.

- Count backward from 347 by 18s as quickly as you can until you fall asleep.

Try these out every night for three to four days. Take notes as to whether it helped you fall asleep faster. If you have some success, continue to use whichever method was more effective.

Embrace Your Inner Scientist

WHY IT WORKS

Our thoughts, feelings, and behaviors are all related.

Let's say your sleep has been poor and you make a mistake at work. You *think,* "My lack of sleep is impacting my work. I could lose my job." This makes you *feel* anxious and experience *physical* reactions like an increased heart rate. Your *behavior* is to get into bed earlier, even though you aren't tired. You barely get any sleep, and the cycle continues.

Changing our thoughts here would change our feelings and behaviors. But sometimes it's hard to believe in the thought change. Try to think like a scientist by testing out whether or not some of the beliefs that are blocking your progress are actually true.

HOW TO DO IT

1. Identify your negative beliefs about sleep. For example, let's say your belief is, "I have a limited amount of energy," which could cause you to be inactive most of the day to preserve your energy.

2. Think of the opposite for each negative belief. The alternative for the above belief would be, "Being inactive increases fatigue."

3. Design small experiments to test out each opposite belief. For the one we developed above, you could alternate between days of being more and less active for two weeks and record how you feel and what your sleep was like every day.

4. At the end of your experiment, you should have gathered enough data to prove that your opposite belief is true.

Plan for Not Sleeping

WHY IT WORKS

The more you lie awake trying to sleep, the less likely it is you'll actually sleep. Anytime you "try" to sleep, you are telling yourself that if you don't sleep, it will be uncomfortable or painful for you the next day. Thoughts like these cause an increase in your level of arousal or anxiety when you need to be calm and relaxed. Over time, your bed becomes associated with anxiety and not sleeping.

It's better not to try to sleep unless you're actually ready.

Plan ahead of time for different things you can do that are both pleasant and not too stimulating when you can't sleep.

1. Write down a list of things you can do in the beginning, middle, or end of your sleep period. Here are some suggestions.

    a. **Beginning:** prepare food for the following day, listen to relaxing music, fold clothes, write, stretch, give yourself a massage

    b. **Middle:** do some light reading, listen to an audiobook, do a puzzle, draw or color, declutter, make your shopping list

    c. **End:** grab something at your favorite coffee shop, watch the sunrise, meditate, go for a walk or workout, tidy up your room, water plants

2. Try each of these out at least once and write down notes the next day about whether they helped.

3. Continue to use the methods that worked the best.

4. Notice that your arousal and negative association with your bed decrease over time.

Practice Mindfulness

WHY IT WORKS

Mindfulness is the act of paying attention to the present moment on purpose and without judgment. Originating from Buddhism, it was brought to the west in the 1960s and later secularized and adapted to treat many physical and mental health difficulties. Research on mindfulness practices has exploded in the last few decades. A recent comprehensive review of numerous studies conducted in the last eight years on the impact of mindfulness on sleep found that mindfulness-based treatments are efficacious for improving symptoms of insomnia when compared to placebo or no treatment at all.

Training yourself to pay attention to the present moment and redirect your attention back to a focal point, repetitively and over time, will allow you to more easily defuse yourself from difficult thoughts or experiences. And that will allow you to be more relaxed and ready for sleep.

Practicing mindfulness is simple, but not easy. Our attention is constantly being pulled in many directions. It's important to embrace patience and non-judgment so you don't get discouraged when starting your practice.

Start with small goals and build your practice slowly—try carving out five minutes in your day two to three times per week. Then, extend your practice by five-minute increments and/or the number of days per week. There are many apps available for download that offer free guided meditations (e.g., Insight Timer, Calm). You can also join a meditation group.

RECOMMENDED APPS FOR SLEEP AND RELAXATION

Many apps can be used in conjunction with sleep strategies. Just remember to turn down the blue light on your devices at least two hours before bedtime.

1. **CBT-i Coach:** Developed by VA's National Center for PTSD, Stanford School of Medicine, and DoD's National Center for Telehealth and Technology, this app provides useful information on sleep and insomnia and can be used to record your sleep and calculate your sleep efficiency.

2. **CBT Thought Diary:** This app allows you to challenge your negative thoughts about sleep. It walks you through how to examine evidence for and against your thoughts and recognize whether you are engaging in cognitive distortions.

3. **Top Mindfulness/Relaxation Apps:** While there are numerous available, the following are the most well-liked by colleagues and clients. Experiment with all to determine which suits you best:
   a. Calm
   b. Insight Timer
   c. Headspace
   d. Stop, Breathe, & Think

Nothing Worthwhile Is Easy

WHY IT WORKS

With the way modern society functions, we're primed to expect immediate responses. If a webpage takes too long to load, we get frustrated. If a friend doesn't reply to our texts quickly, we get confused. If we have to wait in a long line, we get angry. It's no wonder then that when it comes to behavior changes, we expect anything we try to cure our problems instantaneously.

Unfortunately, this is not how change works. Developing patience is essential to your success. It will enable you to ride the wave of any inevitable setbacks you may experience.

HOW TO DO IT

You have most likely been suffering for months, or even years. It's normal and understandable that you'd like things to change quickly. Instead of allowing yourself to get wrapped up in negative or anxious thoughts about your lack of progress, take a deep breath and check in with yourself by reflecting on these questions:

- Is your desire for things to be different making you feel any better?
- Have you learned anything new by having these thoughts?
- Do you think these thoughts will improve your progress?

If you answered no to any of these questions, work on either letting these thoughts go or providing yourself with some words of encouragement instead. Perhaps you could instead say to yourself: "I am having a hard time right now and want things to be better; this is understandable. But with patience and continued practice, my sleep can improve."

Go from Burned Out to Energized Within

WHY IT WORKS

Work emails seem to never stop and our to-do lists appear to be constantly growing. Work environments such as these can lead to high rates of occupational burnout—a state of overwhelming exhaustion, feelings of cynicism and detachment from the job, and a sense of ineffectiveness and lack of accomplishment. If left unaddressed, burnout can contribute to several health consequences, including insomnia.

Ignoring what's causing your burnout will only send you into an insomnia cycle again. It's important that you take a close look at what's contributing to it.

HOW TO DO IT

1. Start with identifying what's contributing to your burnout. This may be very obvious, or you may

have to write out a list of contributing factors. Are you being overworked? Is the company culture or work environment not in line with your values? Is there no opportunity for growth?

2. Are there any steps you can take to change what's contributing to your burnout? Can you talk to your boss about changing your role? Is it time to start saying "no" more often? Are you not using your vacation time? Plan out small steps you can take to work on some of these items.

3. Create a list of your top five values, or what gives your life meaning. Reassess whether your current job is in line with your values. If not, are there steps you can take to change your role? Is it time to consider a career change?

Learn to Be a Yogi

WHY IT WORKS

Originating from ancient India, yoga is a set of physical, mental, and spiritual practices. A recent review of numerous studies examining the effect of mind-body therapies on insomnia found that yoga is an effective treatment for reducing symptoms and improving sleep quality in a variety of populations.

Our mind and body require relaxation to sleep. Yoga encourages the parasympathetic nervous system, otherwise known as the rest-and-digest system, which helps do just that.

HOW TO DO IT

Build a regular yoga practice into your self-care routine. Start with thirty minutes once per week and slowly increase the frequency and duration. There are countless yoga studios as well as instructional videos online (e.g., "Yoga with Adriene" on YouTube). Only gentle and restorative poses should be used close to bedtime.

Stretch It Out:

Here are a few restorative poses to use at night:

- Lie on the floor on your back and place the back of your legs up a wall, keeping them straight. Your body will form an L-shaped pose. Hold this position for several minutes while relaxing your muscles and focusing on your breathing.

- Lie on the floor on your back. Press the soles of your feet together, letting your knees fall to the sides. Hold this pose for about a minute and focus on your breathing.

- Lie on the floor on your back with your legs straight, arms by sides, and palms facing up. Breathe slowly and deeply, focusing on your inhales and exhales.

Challenge Unhelpful Thoughts

WHY IT WORKS

One reason insomnia persists is due to the high levels of arousal or anxiety we feel when we think about all of the potential bad outcomes of not receiving adequate sleep. The more anxious we are, the less likely our body is to produce sleep.

While your distress over your symptoms is certainly justified, actively thinking about it throughout the day (or when you are triggered by something) is most likely not helping you get any better. You can stop this pattern by training yourself to notice when the destructive thinking is happening, and then challenge and eventually change the thoughts.

HOW TO DO IT

Use the thought table to work on challenging your thinking. Start by filling out the first three columns

on a daily basis for one week or until you're better
at noticing your negative thoughts about sleep as
they arise. Next, go through all of the columns by
looking at the factual evidence for and against your
thoughts, coming up with a more helpful alternative,

SITUATION	MOOD	THOUGHTS	
In what situation were you thinking about sleep?	What were you feeling and how intense was it (0% to 100%)?	What were you thinking about?	

and rating your mood after the exercise. You should notice that your anxiety decreases after engaging in this. Practice this daily until the alternative thoughts occur automatically.

	EVIDENCE FOR THOUGHTS	EVIDENCE AGAINST THOUGHTS	ALTERNATIVE THOUGHT	MOOD
	What evidence do you have to support these thoughts (facts only)?	What evidence do you have that does not support these thoughts?	Weighing the evidence for and against, what is a more balanced, helpful thought?	What is your mood now and how intense is it?

Try Sitting Up

WHY IT WORKS

The longer we're awake or anxious in bed, the more our bed becomes associated with those things. To break the association, we must get out of bed every time we aren't asleep. See "Quit *Lying* to Yourself" on page 27 for more information on this strategy.

Getting out of bed every time you're awake won't work for you if the idea of getting out of bed makes you even more anxious; you're a chronic pain sufferer and it isn't realistic for you; you're at risk of falling and hurting yourself; you're too overzealous about getting out of bed; you don't allow yourself enough time in bed to fall back asleep; or you have a fear of the bed due to trauma.

If you fall into any of these categories, you can use a different technique called counter-control therapy, which is nearly as effective as stimulus control. Instead of getting up, you sit up. This is a different position than the one we normally take to sleep, which helps our brain learn lying down is for sleeping and sitting up is for other activities.

HOW TO DO IT

If, to the best of your estimation, it's been twenty minutes and you haven't fallen asleep, sit up in your bed and engage in some type of calming activity like reading or watching an episode of something on TV. This can be more effective for middle of the night awakenings than sleep onset.

SLEEP AND TRAUMA

Experiencing, witnessing, or even learning about traumatic events can leave a person vulnerable to several mental health symptoms, including insomnia.

When we experience trauma, our fight-or-flight system gets activated. It floods our brain with a variety of chemicals designed to keep us awake and "on guard." Trauma can also cause us to experience nightmares or flashbacks.

That hyperarousal can prevent sleep. It can also cause the trauma survivor to avoid sleeping because they might be afraid of having nightmares or being unable to respond to urgent situations.

If you are experiencing any of these symptoms, please know it is very common and is in no way a sign of weakness. You will still benefit greatly from addressing your insomnia symptoms and may even see an improvement in your trauma symptoms. There are also many professionals trained in treating trauma and insomnia who can be an additional source of support.

Stay Awake

WHY IT WORKS

Our body desires homeostasis—steady and stable internal conditions necessary for survival. One function of our homeostatic system is to ensure we're receiving the sleep our brain and body require to function optimally. So, less sleep one night will result in more sleep the next.

The longer time we spend awake, the more our body produces a chemical called adenosine. The more adenosine we have stored, the more we will sleep when given the opportunity. Sleep restriction strategies used in CBT-I take advantage of this principle. Purposefully depriving yourself of an opportunity for sleep for several weeks will allow your body to reset its homeostatic functions.

While this strategy works very well to improve insomnia symptoms, people can have a difficult time following it. One reason is because they have a hard time keeping themselves awake until their scheduled bedtime. See "No Pain, No Gain" on page 69 for information on how to set this.

HOW TO DO IT

After you have determined your time-in-bed prescription and scheduled your bed and rise times, it's time to brainstorm ideas to keep yourself awake. Write down several ideas in one column. In the column next to it, rate the likelihood (low, medium, or high) this idea will keep you awake. In the next column, rate the likelihood this idea will interfere with your sleep. Implement the ideas that have a high likelihood of keeping you awake and a low likelihood of interfering with your sleep.

Take On an Attitude of Gratitude

WHY IT WORKS

Gratitude can produce many positive impacts on our lives. It can also impact our sleep, such that the more grateful we are, the better we sleep at night.

It's thought that the main way gratitude impacts sleep is through a difference in thought patterns, especially before sleep. Many people with insomnia experience negative or worrisome thoughts about a variety of topics before bed. Thoughts like this activate our fight-or-flight response. People who practice gratitude, on the other hand, generally experience a wider array of positive thoughts about the way they perceive their life, allowing them to feel calmer and more content, which causes them to sleep better.

HOW TO DO IT

For at least two weeks, try carving out ten to fifteen minutes of your day to build this practice by starting a gratitude journal.

Get Out Your Pen and Paper:
Although there is no wrong way to do this, here are a few different approaches:

1. Write down five things per day that you're grateful for. These can be people, events, experiences, things—anything. Be specific.
2. Write down three things that went well for you each day. Describe what happened and why you think it went well.
3. Write a letter to a person you are grateful for and/or who helped you in some way, whom you haven't had an opportunity to thank yet.

Create a Bedtime Ritual

WHY IT WORKS

Many of us know routines are helpful for children—they offer structure and stability and often help kids build healthy habits. As adults, we sometimes forget the same benefits apply to us. We can get so wrapped up in the stressors of our daily lives that we skip out on the very behaviors that can help to reduce that stress. The more our stress builds, the lower our chances of producing quality sleep become, leading to a perpetual cycle.

One way to break this cycle is by building healthy sleep routines. Engaging in a set of rituals to help prepare you for sleep can cue your brain that it's time to rest. Because our brain likes short-cuts, the more you repeat a certain behavior over time, the more automatic it becomes. If you achieve relaxation every time you engage in your ritual and are able to fall asleep, after time, engaging in those same rituals will cue your brain to produce sleep automatically.

HOW TO DO IT

Develop your own set of relaxing rituals to engage in at least one hour before your bedtime. Here's an example you can follow:

1. Dim the lights.
2. Turn off all electronic devices or put on blue-light blocking glasses.
3. Take a warm shower or bath.
4. Floss and brush your teeth. Wash your face.
5. Read on the couch until sleepiness emerges. Go to sleep.

Repeat this every day, regardless of where you are, until it becomes automatic. Remember to keep things balanced by watching out for any signs that your ritual has become counterproductive, such as thoughts that you "must" engage in this ritual otherwise you won't sleep at all.

Increase Your Coping

WHY IT WORKS

Imagine you're feeling tired and irritated because you didn't get any sleep the night before. While at work, you make a minor mistake. You might start thinking your insomnia is causing problems at work, which might make you feel even more fatigued and frustrated.

Now, imagine that you're feeling energized and happy because you received adequate sleep. Imagine what you might be thinking now if you make that same mistake. Probably quite the opposite. You might be more inclined to depersonalize the situation, remind yourself that mistakes happen to everyone, and move forward.

When we're upset, it's difficult to access the more balanced, rational thoughts that help us feel better. Writing down helpful statements ahead of time can remind us of other thoughts or coping strategies when we're not able to easily access them in the moment. This helps reduce our overall levels of arousal, stress, and anxiety, which, in turn, helps us sleep.

HOW TO DO IT

1. Think about the moments you experience fatigue, anxiety, frustration, and other negative moods. Now write out the types of thoughts you typically experience that make you feel worse. Next to each of those thoughts, write a more balanced thought that might make you feel better.
2. Write out coping statements on index cards, one per card (e.g., "The chances of losing my job are very low," or "Pause and take deep, slow breaths").
3. Keep these cards with you and review them every time you notice yourself in a negative mood state.

Don't Ignore Concurrent Conditions

WHY IT WORKS

Some of the most common precipitating factors of insomnia are related to family, health, or work/school-related events, particularly those of a negative nature. If these issues are not concurrently addressed along with your insomnia, they can make your recovery more difficult.

Additionally, people who have an insomnia disorder often have other mental health-related diagnoses concurrently. The most frequent mental health disorders that co-occur with insomnia are bipolar, depressive, and anxiety disorders. It is important to treat these other disorders as well, if not even first. Not doing so can delay the improvement of your insomnia symptoms and also negatively contribute to your overall well-being.

If you haven't been able to address the precipitating factors of your insomnia on your own yet, it might be time to consider reaching out to people in your life who you can call on for extra support (e.g., friends, family, partners, clergy members, or mental health professionals).

If a healthcare professional has diagnosed you with a mental health disorder other than insomnia or you suspect you may have one, please don't ignore it. In particular, if you are currently under extreme distress (due to psychological or medical reasons), have an active substance use disorder, bipolar disorder, or panic disorder, these should be addressed prior to the insomnia. Identify a healthcare provider both whom you are comfortable with and who has expertise in the difficulties you are facing.

INSOMNIA AND DEPRESSION

Major Depressive Disorder (MDD) causes an individual to experience depressed mood and/or a loss of interest or pleasure in almost all activities most of the day, nearly every day, for two weeks or more. They also experience several other symptoms (totaling at least five at the same time), one of which may include insomnia.

The mental health community used to believe MDD *caused* insomnia. We now know that untreated insomnia actually leaves an individual with twice the risk of developing MDD and can even predict suicide risk.

For those already suffering from MDD, untreated insomnia makes it less likely they'll be able to recover from their depression, even after receiving treatment for it. If they recover, but the insomnia continues, they have a higher chance of experiencing depression again, which is why it is so important to address both disorders concurrently.

Get Off the Thought Train

WHY IT WORKS

Oftentimes when we experience anxious thoughts, we either get caught up in them or try to push them out because they're uncomfortable. However, doing this can actually make us feel even worse. Getting caught up or tangled with our thoughts can make us feel more out of control, while trying to push our thoughts out can paradoxically make them grow even stronger. However, learning to observe your thoughts as they arise, without adding to them or attempting to push them out, can help reduce your level of stress. This can help you defuse from your thoughts and re-center yourself, allowing you to sleep better.

The next time you notice anxious thoughts about sleep, try the following exercise:

1. Find a comfortable position, either seated or lying down. Close your eyes and picture yourself sitting on a mountaintop. Notice what's around you.

2. Now, imagine a train track stretching across the horizon. Notice a train appear at the end of the track, slowly moving toward the center of your view.

3. Think of each car that goes by as one of your thoughts. Notice each one pass, let it go, and move to the next car.

4. If you notice an urge to jump on any of the cars, gently guide your attention back to where you are—seated calmly on the mountain, observing the train.

5. Continue this practice for several minutes until the urge to jump on the car decreases.

It's Not the Final Countdown

WHY IT WORKS

Ever find yourself checking your clock in the middle of the night after what seems like an eternity of tossing and turning only to find yourself counting down how many more precious hours or minutes you have until the dreaded alarm goes off? The more you think about how little time you have left for sleep, the more pressure you've built to fall back asleep. And pressure puts our brain on high alert, activating our fight-or-flight system, making sleep nearly impossible.

Some people say checking helps them know they still have more time to sleep, which takes the pressure off. While this may work a few times, all you're doing is building a habit to check every time you wake up in the middle of the night. You're bound to have moments when this doesn't work, but you'll still be tempted to do it again because the behavior has been intermittently reinforced.

If you use your cell phone as your alarm, consider purchasing a good old-fashioned alarm clock instead. Keep your cell phone out of sight, and place your alarm clock far away from the bed where it doesn't face you. That way, you'll be much less tempted to turn it around to check.

Everyone wakes up multiple times throughout the night, even good sleepers—they just don't notice it. Learning to tell yourself that it's normal to wake up will decrease your anxiety and help you fall back asleep faster.

Qigong

WHY IT WORKS

Qigong originated in China with roots in Chinese medicine, philosophy, and martial arts. It's a mind-body practice that integrates posture, movement, breathing, sound, and focused intent. A recent study that analyzed several randomized clinical trials found that qigong showed significant effects on improving sleep quality.

Qigong regulates body functions through slow, gentle movements, regulated breathing, and mindful concentration, which also promotes circulation. Practicing qigong lowers stress and anxiety, improving sleep.

HOW TO DO IT

Carve out about five to ten minutes of time three to four times per week, ideally in the morning or afternoon. There are instructional videos available for free online (e.g., "Qigong for Vitality"), but here's one five-minute exercise to get you started if your body allows it:

1. Standing (or sitting upright) with your feet shoulder-width apart and your knees slightly bent, extend your arms out and upward toward the sky with your palms facing up, forming a big circle with your arms.

2. Move your palms toward each other and let your hands float down through the midline of your body.

3. Repeat this motion, taking a deep breath in as your hands circle upward and breathing out as your hands float down through the midline of your body to your lower abdomen.

4. Do this for a few minutes, focusing on your breathing, and releasing any tension as your hands move downward.

Once you've finished, check in with your mind and body. Do you feel more relaxed?

Believe in Yourself

WHY IT WORKS

Your belief in your *ability* to deal with new tasks or difficulties, otherwise known as self-efficacy, can actually determine whether you are successful in accomplishing that task or overcoming that hurdle. If you're trying to improve your insomnia, but deep down you believe that you won't be able to, then any expected or normal setback you experience will reinforce that belief. You'll be more inclined to give up.

Self-efficacy develops through performing tasks successfully, adequately coping with any challenges, witnessing others (especially those similar to ourselves) successfully complete tasks, receiving positive reinforcement or words of encouragement about our ability to succeed, and our own emotional states or physical reactions to certain situations.

Here are some ways to improve your self-efficacy:

1. Every day you're successful in accomplishing at least one of the strategies in this book, write it down. Celebrate your success by providing yourself words of encouragement or praise.

2. Tell a close friend, family member, or confidant who is likely to be a source of support and encouragement about the goals you've set. Kindly ask them to check in with you weekly, providing you with praise for whatever you were able to accomplish—even if it was only one thing.

3. Any time you experience a setback, notice what you say to yourself. If it's negative or discouraging, think about what you'd say to a good friend who was in the same situation, and say it to yourself.

Put Your Own Mask on First

WHY IT WORKS

Many of us struggle with chronic stress due to numerous responsibilities piling up. It can be very easy to put ourselves last on our list of priorities. While this sometimes can't be helped, constantly putting our needs last can make it harder for us to take care of our other responsibilities in the long run. If you've ever been on an airplane, you've probably heard the safety instructions to put your own oxygen mask on first, before you help others. The same applies to our daily life—if we don't take care of ourselves, there is no way we can take care of all the other things that need our attention.

Spend time identifying a self-care plan you can practice daily for at least fifteen minutes by writing down responses to the following questions:

1. What are some things I can do to be kind to my mind and body?

    a. Examples: stretch, engage in deep breathing, drink water, get a massage, go for a walk outdoors, practice mindfulness

2. What hobbies or activities do I enjoy engaging in that I know produce pleasure or joy?

    a. Examples: being in nature, hiking, going to the beach, listening to music, learning a new skill, watching movies, reading, traveling, cooking

3. Who can I count on to be sources of support if I need someone to talk to or be present with me?

    a. Examples: friends, family, members in a support group, mentors, pets

ALEX'S SLEEP STORY

When I asked Alex what brought him to my office, he told me about the years of grueling hours he had put into perfecting the skills he needed to excel in his career. After overcoming several professional hurdles, he was given a promotion.

Shortly after receiving it, he found himself lying in bed unable to drown out his thoughts. Riddled with doubt about his new role, his sleep grew increasingly worse over the past six months. One day, he noticed that he made an error on an important assignment. "I can't lose my job," he told me as his eyes welled with tears.

With time, we uncovered how his anxiety surrounding his new role contributed to an inability to decompress from work.

We started a stimulus control and self-care plan.

Alex's ability to change the behaviors that were maintaining his symptoms enabled him to break free from his insomnia cycle.

Work Through Your Worries

WHY IT WORKS

Our brain remembers unfinished tasks more than finished ones. This causes a buildup of tension that induces a need to complete that unfinished task, known as the Zeigarnik effect. If we stop working on a task or don't experience closure, especially before bedtime, our brain keeps that issue active in our mind in order to produce enough energy to finish it.

Researchers have found that engaging in a form of constructive worry where the individual takes active steps toward finding solutions to their issues well before bedtime, can actually reduce levels of cognitive arousal. Then, our minds can settle down and we can sleep.

HOW TO DO IT

1. For the next week, find a fifteen-minute period to spend time on this strategy at least three to four hours before bedtime and after most of your tasks are finished for the day.

2. Take out a sheet of paper and fold it in half, making two columns.

3. On one side of the sheet, write down a few major issues or tasks that are likely to keep you up at night.

4. On the other side of the sheet, write down at least one immediate step you can take toward solving each problem.

5. When you're finished, fold it in half and set it aside. Every time you catch yourself worrying about the same problems in the middle of the night, remind yourself that there is nothing more you can do in this moment.

A Bedtime Snack

WHY IT WORKS

Hunger can keep you awake. From an evolutionary perspective, this makes sense. If we were hungry, our brain needed to be awake and alert enough to go find food in order to survive. Plus, being very hungry can feel downright painful, which can prevent us from falling asleep.

Research suggests that the two metabolic hormones called leptin and ghrelin are responsible for this effect. When we consume food, leptin communicates to our brain that we are satisfied. Ghrelin, on the other hand, communicates hunger. Having enough leptin to suppress the secretion of ghrelin will allow us to sleep throughout the night without being awakened by hunger.

Although it is better to avoid heavy meals before bedtime, being hungry won't help us either. Therefore, it's best to maintain a balance of not eating too much too late, but also making sure our stomach is

full enough that it will not keep us awake throughout the night.

HOW TO DO IT

If you notice you are hungry before bedtime, try
consuming a small snack with protein in it, as
protein contains tryptophan, which will stimulate
melatonin production in our brain—the hormone
responsible for our sleep drive. Just remember to
avoid foods containing caffeine (like chocolate)
and spicy, acidic, high-fat, and sugary foods before
bedtime. See "Food for Sleep" on page 109 for more
information.

Here are some bedtime snack suggestions:

- Milk
- Peanut butter
- Cheese

Tai Chi

WHY IT WORKS

Originating in China, tai chi is a gentle physical exercise and meditation that involves a series of movements practiced in a slow, attentive manner along with deep breathing. An analysis of a dozen randomized control trials conducted on the impact of tai chi on insomnia found that it improves sleep quality in a variety of populations.

One tai chi style in particular, called Tai Chi Chih (TCC), has been found to be just as effective in treating insomnia as CBT-I when practiced weekly for three months. Developed by Justin Stone in the 1970s, TCC consists of nineteen movements and one pose focused on circulating and balancing the body's energy. It's thought to improve insomnia symptoms by teaching people control over physical functioning and levels of arousal through mindful movement that emphasizes the connection between mind and body.

TCC is generally safe for people of all ages and fitness levels, as it's low impact and puts minimal stress on muscles and joints. Modification or avoidance of certain postures may be recommended for people with certain conditions (e.g., severe osteoporosis, fractures, back pain).

While you can learn TCC through books or videos (such as *T'ai Chi Chih! Joy Thru Movement* by Justin Stone), it may be helpful to work with a certified teacher at first. Start with carving out ten minutes per day to learn the different movements, and increase your time once you're successful.

Keep It Dark

WHY IT WORKS

All light is sensed through our eyes, which sends signals to different areas of our brain, including the suprachiasmatic nucleus (SCN). The SCN is responsible for the timing of when we're awake or asleep. When it receives light signals, it communicates to our brain that it's daytime, even if we're only being exposed to artificial light from lamps or electronic devices.

Researchers have confirmed this effect, finding that light in the bedroom significantly suppresses melatonin levels and shortens the amount of time we sleep. Interestingly, our eyes do not need to be open for this communication to occur. So, if we've turned off all the lights in our bedroom and closed our eyes, but there's still light peering in through our window or from another room, it will keep us awake/wake us up. This is why it's important to block out as much light as possible in our bedrooms throughout our sleep period.

HOW TO DO IT

- Inspect your bedroom for any sources of artificial light, like alarm clocks, light coming in through your window, electronic devices, or even the power button from the TV.

- Block these sources of light—try blackout shades or curtains for the window and turn around other sources of light or cover them with a piece of cloth.

- If you're worried you might not be able to make your way to the bathroom safely, try placing a very dim night light in your bathroom.

Don't Stress, Compress

WHY IT WORKS

Although sleep restriction works very well if you're able to implement it, some people experience difficulty putting it into practice—generally those with high anxiety about sleep, who may have thoughts about not being able to tolerate restriction. For this reason, an alternative form of sleep restriction, called sleep compression, was developed.

Instead of drastically restricting your time in bed and building it back up, compression does the opposite—gradually restricting your time in bed in thirty-minute increments until your sleep normalizes. While this strategy is equally effective in treating insomnia, it's a much slower process. Patience will be essential to your progress. This strategy is also helpful for those in which restriction is contraindicated (i.e., those with bipolar or panic disorder).

1. Use a sleep diary (like the "CBT-i Coach" app, or the one on page 22) to record your sleep for a one- to two-week period and determine your average time in bed (TIB).

2. Subtract thirty minutes from your average TIB to determine your prescribed TIB.

3. Set a consistent rise time based on your schedule, chronotype, and TIB prescription. Stick to this for one week and continue to record your sleep.

4. Reduce your TIB every week for thirty minutes while maintaining a consistent rise time until your sleep normalizes. Here, that means once the percentage of your average TIB to total sleep time (sleep efficiency) is over 90%, or you start to feel sleepy during the day.

RELAPSE PREVENTION

After trying the strategies in this book, you should be able to identify which work best for you in finding relief from your insomnia symptoms. Now you'll know how to address your insomnia symptoms if they ever resurface in the future. Be proactive and make a list of the strategies that worked so that you can easily remind yourself what to do if your insomnia ever returns, well before your symptoms grow worse.

After you've experienced relief, consider writing yourself a letter about your journey with insomnia, as well as how you were able to improve your symptoms. Add in some words of encouragement or comfort should you ever experience difficulties in the future. If you can't think of your own, you can borrow these words from me: You got through this before, and you can definitely do it again!

Resources

BOOKS

Carney, Colleen, and Rachel Manber (2009). *Quiet Your Mind and Get to Sleep: Solutions to Insomnia for Those with Depression, Anxiety, or Chronic Pain.* Oakland: New Harbinger.

Edinger, Jack D., and Colleen E. Carney (2014). *Overcoming Insomnia: A Cognitive-Behavioral Therapy Approach Workbook.* New York: Oxford University Press.

Hauri, Peter J., and Shirley Linde (1996). *No More Sleepless Nights.* New York: John Wiley and Sons.

Jacobs, Gregg D. (2009). *Say Goodnight to Insomnia: The Six-Week, Drug-Free Program Developed at Harvard Medical School.* New York: Henry Holt.

Stone, Justin (2009). *T'ai Chi Chih! Joy Thru Movement.* Good Karma Press.

WEBSITES

Automated Morningness-Eveningness Questionnaire (AutoMEQ): http://www.cet-surveys.com/index .php?sid=61524

CBT for Insomnia Provider Directory: https://cbti .directory/index.php/search-for-a-provider

CBT-i Coach app: https://apps.apple.com/ca/app /cbt-i-coach/id655918660 and https://play.google .com/store/apps/details?id=gov.va.mobilehealth .ncptsd.cbti

Insomnia Severity Index: https://www.myhealth .va.gov/mhv-portal-web/web/myhealthevet /insomnia-severity-index1

Mayo Clinic BMI Calculator: https://www .mayoclinic.org/diseases-conditions/obesity /in-depth/bmi-calculator/itt-20084938

Progressive Muscle Relaxation: https://www.youtube .com/watch?v=1nZEdqcGVzo

Qigong for Vitality: https://www.qigongforvitality.com/

STOP-Bang Questionnaire to assess sleep apnea: http://www.stopbang.ca/osa/screening.php

UCLA Mindful Awareness Research Center Free Guided Meditations: https://www.uclahealth.org/marc/mindful-meditations

Yoga with Adriene: https://www.youtube.com/user/yogawithadriene

References

Aeschbach, D., Sher, L., Postolache, T. T., Matthews, J. R., Jackson, M. A., & Wehr, T. A. (2003). A longer biological night in long sleepers than in short sleepers. *The Journal of Clinical Endocrinology & Metabolism, 88*(1), 26–30. https://doi.org/10.1210/jc.2002-020827

American Psychiatric Association (2013). *Diagnostic And Statistical Manual of Mental Disorders, Fifth Edition.* Washington, DC.

Angarita, G. A., Emadi, N., Hodges, S., & Morgan, P. T. (2016). Sleep abnormalities associated with alcohol, cannabis, cocaine, and opiate use: A comprehensive review. *Addiction Science & Clinical Practice, 11*(1), 9. https://doi.org/10.1186/s13722-016-0056-7

Babson, K. A., Sottile, J., & Morabito, D. (2017). Cannabis, Cannabinoids, and Sleep: A Review of the Literature. *Current Psychiatry Reports, 19*(4). https://doi.org/10.1007/s11920-017-0775-9

Baglioni, C., Battagliese, G., Feige, B., Spiegelhalder, K., Nissen, C., Voderholzer, U., . . . Riemann, D. (2011). Insomnia as a predictor of depression: A meta-analytic evaluation of longitudinal epidemiological studies. *Journal of Affective Disorders, 135*(1–3), 10–19. https://doi.org/10.1016/j.jad.2011.01.011

Ballesio, A., Aquino, M. R. J. V, Kyle, S. D., Ferlazzo, F., & Lombardo, C. (2019). Executive functions in insomnia disorder: A systematic review and exploratory meta-analysis. *Frontiers in Psychology, 10*, 101. https://doi.org/10.3389/fpsyg.2019.00101

Bandura, A. (1977). Self-efficacy: Toward a unifying theory of behavioral change. *Psychological Review, 84*(2), 191–215. https://doi.org/10.1037/0033-295X.84.2.191

Basner, M., Babisch, W., Davis, A., Brink, M., Clark, C., Janssen, S., & Stansfeld, S. (2014). Auditory and non-auditory effects of noise on health. *The Lancet, 383*(9925), 1325–32. https://doi.org/10.1016/S0140-6736(13)61613-X

Bastien, C. H., Vallieres, A., & Morin, C. M. (2004). Precipitating factors of insomnia. *Behavioral Sleep Medicine, 2*(1), 50–62. https://doi.org/10.1207/s15402010bsm0201_5

Bernert, R. A., & Nadorff, M. R. (2015). Sleep disturbances and suicide risk. *Sleep Medicine Clinics, 10*(1), 35–9. https://doi.org/10.1016/j.jsmc.2014.11.004

Bootzin, R. R., & Rider, S. P. (1997). Behavioral techniques and biofeedback for insomnia. In *Understanding Sleep: The Evaluation and Treatment of Sleep Disorders,* 315–38. https://doi.org/10.1037/10233-016

Broomfield, N. M., & Espie, C. A. (2003). Initial Insomnia and paradoxical intention: An experimental investigation of putative mechanisms using subjective and actigraphic measurement of sleep. *Behavioural and Cognitive Psychotherapy, 31*(3), 313—24. https://doi.org/10.1017/S1352465803003060

Bubu, O. M., Brannick, M., Mortimer, J., Umasabor-Bubu, O., Sebastião, Y. V., Wen, Y., . . . Anderson, W. M. (2017). Sleep, cognitive impairment, and Alzheimer's disease: a systematic review and meta-analysis. *Sleep, 40*(1), zsw032. https://doi.org/10.1093/sleep/zsw032

Buysse, D. J., Angst, J., Gamma, A., Ajdacic, V., Eich, D., & Rössler, W. (2008). Prevalence, course, and comorbidity of insomnia and depression in young

Adults. *Sleep, 31*(4), 473–80. https://doi.org/10.1093
/sleep/31.4.473

Cappuccio, F. P., Taggart, F. M., Kandala, N.-B., Currie,
A., Peile, E., Stranges, S., & Miller, M. A. (2008).
Meta-analysis of short sleep duration and obesity in
children and adults. *Sleep, 31*(5), 619–26. https://doi
.org/10.1093/sleep/31.5.619

Carney, C. E., & Waters, W. F. (2006). Effects of a
structured problem-solving procedure on pre-sleep
cognitive arousal in college students with insomnia.
Behavioral Sleep Medicine, 4(1), 13–28. https://doi
.org/10.1207/s15402010bsm0401_2

Chang, A.-M., Aeschbach, D., Duffy, J. F., & Czeisler,
C. A. (2015). Evening use of light-emitting eReaders
negatively affects sleep, circadian timing, and
next-morning alertness. *Proceedings of the National
Academy of Sciences of the United States of America,
112*(4), 1232–7. https://doi.org/10.1073/pnas.1418490112

Chung, F., Yegneswaran, B., Liao, P., Chung, S. A., Vaira-
vanathan, S., Islam, S., . . . Shapiro, C. M. (2008). STOP
questionnaire. *Anesthesiology, 108*(5), 812–21.
https://doi.org/10.1097/ALN.0b013e31816d83e4

Conroy, D. A., Kurth, M. E., Strong, D. R., Brower, K. J., & Stein, M. D. (2016). Marijuana use patterns and sleep among community-based young adults. *Journal of Addictive Diseases, 35*(2), 135–43. https://doi.org/10.1080/10550887.2015.1132986

Daley, M., Morin, C. M., LeBlanc, M., Grégoire, J. P., Savard, J., & Baillargeon, L. (2009). Insomnia and its relationship to health-care utilization, work absenteeism, productivity and accidents. *Sleep Medicine, 10*(4), 427–38. https://doi.org/10.1016/j.sleep.2008.04.005

Davies, R., Lacks, P., Storandt, M., & Bertelson, A. D. (1986). Countercontrol treatment of sleep-maintenance insomnia in relation to age. *Psychology and Aging, 1*(3), 233–8. Retrieved from http://www.ncbi.nlm.nih.gov/pubmed/3267403

Driver, H. S., & Taylor, S. R. (2000). Exercise and sleep. *Sleep Medicine Reviews, 4*(4), 387–402. https://doi.org/10.1053/SMRV.2000.0110

Emmons, R. A., & McCullough, M. E. (2003). Counting blessings versus burdens: An experimental investigation of gratitude and subjective well-being in daily life. *Journal of Personality and Social Psychology, 84*(2),

377–89. Retrieved from http://www.ncbi.nlm.nih.gov/pubmed/12585811

Exelmans, L., & Van den Bulck, J. (2017). Bedtime, shuteye time and electronic media: Sleep displacement is a two-step process. *Journal of Sleep Research, 26*(3), 364–70. https://doi.org/10.1111/jsr.12510

Ford, D. E., & Kamerow, D. B. (1989). Epidemiologic study of sleep disturbances and psychiatric disorders. An opportunity for prevention? *JAMA, 262*(11), 1479–84. Retrieved from http://www.ncbi.nlm.nih.gov/pubmed/2769898

Gates, P. J., Albertella, L., & Copeland, J. (2014). The effects of cannabinoid administration on sleep: A systematic review of human studies. *Sleep Medicine Reviews, 18*(6), 477–87. https://doi.org/10.1016/j.smrv.2014.02.005

Gooley, J. J., Chamberlain, K., Smith, K. A., Khalsa, S. B. S., Rajaratnam, S. M. W., Van Reen, E., . . . Lockley, S. W. (2011). Exposure to room light before bedtime suppresses melatonin onset and shortens melatonin duration in humans. *The Journal of Clinical Endocrinology & Metabolism, 96*(3), E463–72. https://doi.org/10.1210/jc.2010-2098

Greer, S. M., Goldstein, A. N., & Walker, M. P. (2013). The impact of sleep deprivation on food desire in the human brain. *Nature Communications, 4*, 2259. https://doi.org/10.1038/NCOMMS3259

Harvey, A. G., & Farrell, C. (2003). The efficacy of a Pennebaker-like writing intervention for poor sleepers. *Behavioral Sleep Medicine, 1*(2), 115–24. https://doi.org/10.1207/S15402010BSM0102_4

Harvey, A. G., & Payne, S. (2002). The management of unwanted pre-sleep thoughts in insomnia: Distraction with imagery versus general distraction. *Behaviour Research and Therapy, 40*(3), 267–77. Retrieved from http://www.ncbi.nlm.nih.gov/pubmed/11863237

Horne, J., & Moore, V. (1985). Sleep EEG effects of exercise with and without additional body cooling. *Electroencephalography and Clinical Neurophysiology, 60*(1), 33–8. https://doi.org/10.1016/0013-4694(85)90948-4

Huedo-Medina, T. B., Kirsch, I., Middlemass, J., Klonizakis, M., & Siriwardena, A. N. (2012). Effectiveness of non-benzodiazepine hypnotics in treatment of adult insomnia: Meta-analysis of data submitted to the Food and Drug Administration. *BMJ (Clinical Research Ed.), 345*, e8343. https://doi.org/10.1136/bmj.e8343

Irwin, M. R., Olmstead, R., Carrillo, C., Sadeghi, N., Nicassio, P., Ganz, P. A., & Bower, J. E. (2017). Tai Chi Chih compared with cognitive behavioral therapy for the treatment of insomnia in survivors of breast cancer: A randomized, partially blinded, noninferiority trial. *Journal of Clinical Oncology, 35*(23), 2656–65. https://doi.org/10.1200/JCO.2016.71.0285

Jackowska, M., Brown, J., Ronaldson, A., & Steptoe, A. (2016). The impact of a brief gratitude intervention on subjective well-being, biology and sleep. *Journal of Health Psychology, 21*(10), 2207–17. https://doi.org/10.1177/1359105315572455

Jaehne, A., Loessl, B., Bárkai, Z., Riemann, D., & Hornyak, M. (2009). Effects of nicotine on sleep during consumption, withdrawal and replacement therapy. *Sleep Medicine Reviews, 13*(5), 363–77. https://doi.org/10.1016/J.SMRV.2008.12.003

Jarrin, D. C., Alvaro, P. K., Bouchard, M.-A., Jarrin, S. D., Drake, C. L., & Morin, C. M. (2018). Insomnia and hypertension: A systematic review. *Sleep Medicine Reviews, 41*, 3–38. https://doi.org/10.1016/J.SMRV.2018.02.003

Kabat-Zinn, J. (2009). *Full Catastrophe Living: Using the Wisdom of Your Body and Mind to Face Stress, Pain, and Illness.* New York: Bantam Dell.

Karp, J. F., Buysse, D. J., Houck, P. R., Cherry, C., Kupfer, D. J., & Frank, E. (2004). Relationship of variability in residual symptoms with recurrence of major depressive disorder during maintenance treatment. *American Journal of Psychiatry, 161*(10), 1877–84. https://doi.org/10.1176/ajp.161.10.1877

Kripke, D. F., Langer, R. D., & Kline, L. E. (2012). Hypnotics' association with mortality or cancer: A matched cohort study. *BMJ Open, 2*(1), e000850. https://doi.org/10.1136/bmjopen-2012-000850

Laugsand, L. E., Vatten, L. J., Platou, C., & Janszky, I. (2011). Insomnia and the risk of acute myocardial infarction. *Circulation, 124*(19), 2073–81. https://doi.org/10.1161/CIRCULATIONAHA.111.025858

Levenson, J. C., Shensa, A., Sidani, J. E., Colditz, J. B., & Primack, B. A. (2016). The association between social media use and sleep disturbance among young adults. *Preventive Medicine, 85*, 36—41. https://doi.org/10.1016/j.ypmed.2016.01.001

Li, F., Fisher, K. J., Harmer, P., Irbe, D., Tearse, R. G., & Weimer, C. (2004). Tai Chi and self-rated quality of sleep and daytime sleepiness in older adults: A randomized controlled trial. *Journal of the American Geriatrics Society, 52*(6), 892–900. https://doi.org/10.1111 /j.1532-5415.2004.52255.x

Lichstein, K. L., Riedel, B. W., Wilson, N. M., Lester, K. W., & Aguillard, R. N. (2001). Relaxation and sleep compression for late-life insomnia: A placebo-controlled trial. *Journal of Consulting and Clinical Psychology, 69*(2), 227–39. Retrieved from http://www.ncbi.nlm.nih .gov/pubmed/11393600

Ma, X., Yue, Z.-Q., Gong, Z.-Q., Zhang, H., Duan, N.-Y., Shi, Y.-T., . . . Li, Y.-F. (2017). The effect of diaphragmatic breathing on attention, negative affect and stress in healthy adults. *Frontiers in Psychology, 8*, 874. https://doi.org/10.3389/fpsyg.2017.00874

McEwen, B. S. (2004). Protection and damage from acute and chronic stress: Allostasis and allostatic overload and relevance to the pathophysiology of psychiatric disorders. *Annals of the New York Academy of Sciences, 1032*(1), 1–7. https://doi.org /10.1196/annals.1314.001

Mitchell, M. D., Gehrman, P., Perlis, M., & Umscheid, C. A. (2012). Comparative effectiveness of cognitive behavioral therapy for insomnia: A systematic review. *BMC Family Practice, 13*(1), 40. https://doi.org/10.1186/1471-2296-13-40

Muzet, A. (2007). Environmental noise, sleep and health. *Sleep Medicine Reviews, 11*(2), 135–42. https://doi.org/10.1016/J.SMRV.2006.09.001

Ohayon, M. M. (2002). Epidemiology of insomnia: What we know and what we still need to learn. *Sleep Medicine Reviews, 6*(2), 97–111. Retrieved from http://www.ncbi.nlm.nih.gov/pubmed/12531146

Pennebaker, J. W. (1997). Writing about emotional experiences as a therapeutic process. *Psychological Science, 8*(3), 162–6. https://doi.org/10.1111/j.1467-9280.1997.tb00403.x

Qaseem, A., Kansagara, D., Forciea, M. A., Cooke, M., & Denberg, T. D. (2016). Management of chronic insomnia disorder in adults: A clinical practice guideline from the american college of physicians. *Annals of Internal Medicine, 165*(2), 125. https://doi.org/10.7326/M15-2175

Rash, J. A., Kavanagh, V. A. J., & Garland, S. N. (2019). A meta-analysis of mindfulness-based therapies for insomnia and sleep disturbance: Moving towards processes of change. *Sleep Medicine Clinics, 14*(2), 209–33. https://doi.org/10.1016/J.JSMC.2019.01.004

Roth, T., Jaeger, S., Jin, R., Kalsekar, A., Stang, P. E., & Kessler, R. C. (2006). Sleep problems, comorbid mental disorders, and role functioning in the national comorbidity survey replication. *Biological Psychiatry, 60*(12), 1364–71. https://doi.org/10.1016/j.biopsych.2006.05.039

Stone, J. F. (1996). *T'ai chi chih!: Joy through movement.* Albuquerque, NM: Good Karma Publishing, Inc.

Sung, E. J., & Tochihara, Y. (2000). Effects of bathing and hot footbath on sleep in winter. *Journal of Physiological Anthropology and Applied Human Science, 19*(1), 21–7. Retrieved from http://www.ncbi.nlm.nih.gov/pubmed/10979246

Trauer, J. M., Qian, M. Y., Doyle, J. S., Rajaratnam, S. M. W., & Cunnington, D. (2015). Cognitive behavioral therapy for chronic insomnia: A systematic review and meta-analysis. *Annals of Internal Medicine, 163*(3), 191–204. https://doi.org/10.7326/M14-2841

Troxel, W. M., Kupfer, D. J., Reynolds III, C. F., Frank, E., Thase, M. E., Miewald, J. M., & Buysse, D. J. (2012). Insomnia and objectively measured sleep disturbances predict treatment outcome in depressed patients treated with psychotherapy or psychotherapy-pharmacotherapy combinations. *The Journal of Clinical Psychiatry, 73*(04), 478–85. https://doi.org/10.4088/JCP.11m07184

Vgontzas, A. N., Liao, D., Pejovic, S., Calhoun, S., Karataraki, M., & Bixler, E. O. (2009). Insomnia with objective short sleep duration is associated with type 2 diabetes: A population-based study. *Diabetes Care, 32*(11), 1980–85. https://doi.org/10.2337/dc09-0284

Vgontzas, A. N., Tsigos, C., Bixler, E. O., Stratakis, C. A., Zachman, K., Kales, A., . . . Chrousos, G. P. (1998). Chronic insomnia and activity of the stress system: A preliminary study. *Journal of Psychosomatic Research, 45*(1), 21–31. https://doi.org/10.1016/S0022-3999(97)00302-4

Wang, X., Li, P., Pan, C., Dai, L., Wu, Y., & Deng, Y. (2019). The effect of mind-body therapies on insomnia: A systematic review and meta-analysis. *Evidence-Based Complementary and Alternative Medicine,* 2019, 1–17. https://doi.org/10.1155/2019/9359807

Waters, W. F., Hurry, M. J., Binks, P. G., Carney, C. E., Lajos, L. E., Fuller, K. H., . . . Tucci, J. M. (2003). Behavioral and hypnotic treatments for insomnia subtypes. *Behavioral Sleep Medicine, 1*(2), 81–101. https://doi.org/10.1207/S15402010BSM0102_2

Watkins, E. R., Mullan, E., Wingrove, J., Rimes, K., Steiner, H., Bathurst, N., . . . Scott, J. (2011). Rumination-focused cognitive-behavioural therapy for residual depression: Phase II randomised controlled trial. *The British Journal of Psychiatry, 199*, 1–6. https://doi.org/10.1192/bjp.bp.110.090282

Wetter, D. W., & Young, T. B. (1994). The relation between cigarette smoking and sleep disturbance. *Preventive Medicine, 23*(3), 328–34. https://doi.org/10.1006/PMED.1994.1046

Wood, A. M., Joseph, S., Lloyd, J., & Atkins, S. (2009). Gratitude influences sleep through the mechanism of pre-sleep cognitions. *Journal of Psychosomatic Research, 66*(1), 43–8. https://doi.org/10.1016/J.JPSYCHORES.2008.09.002

Woodyard, C. (2011). Exploring the therapeutic effects of yoga and its ability to increase quality of life.

International Journal of Yoga, 4(2), 49–54.
https://doi.org/10.4103/0973-6131.85485

Woznica, A. A., Carney, C. E., Kuo, J. R., & Moss, T. G.
(2015). The insomnia and suicide link: Toward an
enhanced understanding of this relationship. *Sleep
Medicine Reviews, 22*, 37–46. https://doi.org/10.1016
/j.smrv.2014.10.004

Wright, K. M., Britt, T. W., Bliese, P. D., Adler, A. B.,
Picchioni, D., & Moore, D. (2011). Insomnia as predictor
versus outcome of PTSD and depression among Iraq
combat veterans. *Journal of Clinical Psychology,
67*(12), 1240–1258. https://doi.org/10.1002/jclp.20845

Yang, P.-Y., Ho, K.-H., Chen, H.-C., & Chien, M.-Y. (2012).
Exercise training improves sleep quality in middle-aged
and older adults with sleep problems: A systematic
review. *Journal of Physiotherapy, 58*(3), 157–63.
https://doi.org/10.1016/S1836-9553(12)70106-6

Youngstedt, S. D., O'Connor, P. J., & Dishman, R. K.
(1997). The effects of acute exercise on sleep: A
quantitative synthesis. *Sleep, 20*(3), 203–14. Retrieved
from http://www.ncbi.nlm.nih.gov/pubmed/9178916

Index

Acknowledgments

I would like to express my sincere gratitude to my publisher, Callisto Media, for giving me the opportunity to write this book, and my editors, Lia Ottaviano and Sara Kendall, for their continual encouragement and sage guidance. I would also like to thank all of the researchers whose immense contributions to the fields of sleep, health, and psychology have advanced the knowledge on the best available treatments for insomnia.

I would not be the psychologist I am today without my mentor, Dr. Shelly Harrell. Thank you for always being a source of inspiration and for your continual guidance and never-ending support throughout the years. To all my clients whom I have had the privilege of providing therapy throughout the years, thank you for allowing me to be a part of your journey and contributing to my purpose. Most importantly, I would like to thank my loving and caring husband, Salar, for his constant support and devotion, and my sister, Rebecca, for her love and friendship. This book would not have been possible without them.

About the Author

 Dr. Nicole Moshfegh is an attending psychologist at the David Geffen School of Medicine at the University of California Los Angeles (UCLA), where she provides psychotherapy and psychodiagnostic assessments for sleep, mood, anxiety, and trauma-related disorders, leads research on physician well-being, and provides teaching and supervision to trainees. She is additionally an adjunct professor at Pepperdine University in the Graduate School of Education and Psychology and is credentialed as a clinical and health service psychologist. She completed her clinical internship and postdoctoral fellowships at UCLA and received her doctoral and master's degrees from Pepperdine University in clinical psychology. Dr. Moshfegh has published and presented at conferences in the areas of multicultural competence, well-being, resilience, mindfulness-based interventions, and major mental illness. She has a private practice in Los Angeles, California, where she provides cognitive-behavioral and mindfulness-based interventions for the treatment of insomnia, anxiety, and mood disorders.

CPSIA information can be obtained
at www.ICGtesting.com
Printed in the USA
LVHW070553220919
631794LV00008B/5/P